The Busy Guide to Food Allergies

Everything you need to know about managing cow's milk allergy and other childhood food allergies

Zoe T. Williams

Orders: Please contact www.myallergykitchen.com or email
zoe@myallergykitchen.com

First Published: 2019

Copyright © 2019 Zoe T. Williams

The moral rights of the author have been asserted.

All rights reserved. Apart from any permitted use under UK copyright
law, no part of this publication may be reproduced or transmitted in any
form or by any means, electronic or mechanical, including photocopying,
recording or any information, storage or retrieval system, without
permission in writing from the publisher or under licence from the
Copyrights Licensing Agency Limited. Further details of such licenses
(for reprographic reproduction) may be obtained from the Copyright
Licensing Agency Ltd, Barnard's Inn, 86 Fetter Lane, London EC4A 1EN

ISBN-13: 978-1-7311-3256-7

Although the author has made every effort to ensure that the information in this book was correct at the time of publication, the author does not assume and hereby disclaims any liability to any party for any loss, damage or disruption caused by errors or omissions, whether such errors or omissions result from negligence, accident, or any other cause.

This book is not intended as a substitute for the medical advice of a qualified health professional. No information in this book should be relied upon to determine diet, make a medical diagnosis, or determine treatment for a medical condition.

CONTENTS

ACKNOWLEDGMENTS

I would like to thank my husband Chris for his unwavering support as I have written this book. He is my best friend and supports me in all my endeavours.

To my youngest daughter Ellie – she is the reason why this book exists.

To my eldest daughter Kayleigh who is a great advocate for those with allergies, including her sister.

To everyone who has contacted me via social media or email. I think it's so important for us all to support and learn from each other along the way. The doctors may know the science behind it all but we are the experts on bringing up children with allergies.

To all my friends who have encouraged me along the way.

To all the other parents on the CMPA Support groups on Facebook who have answered my questions as we have been learning and overcoming problems related to our daughter's food allergies on our own allergy journey.

WELCOME

I am so happy to be able to bring you this book about managing your child's food allergies. The contents of this book are based on my experience of bringing up my young daughter who has multiple food allergies, speaking to other parents of children with food allergies, and countless hours of research. I hope that by putting everything I have learned into this book, I can help other parents who are going through the same thing. I have written the book that would have helped me when we first started to realise that my daughter had allergies, and I hope that it will help you too.

In my personal experience, there is very little practical help and support for people with food allergies. There is no cure (yet) and so medical support is very limited. A doctor can help you diagnose food allergies and prescribe emergency medication, and a dietitian can give you information about foods to avoid and nutrition, but this doesn't help you with the day-to-day problems like 'Will my child be safe at nursery or school?', 'How can we go on holiday?' or 'How do I talk to my child about their allergies?'. This book has been designed to fill that gap.

I think the first 6 – 12 months of the food allergy 'journey' is the most difficult time. Getting a diagnosis can months, while you wait for referrals and test results or work through an exclusion diet. There is a lot of uncertainty. Then once you know what your child's allergies are, you have to learn which specific foods they can and can't eat. This involves a lot of adjustment and affects the whole family. You also have to learn how to do everyday things differently. You will need to change how you shop, cook and store food. For things like eating out, travelling and social events there is a lot more planning and preparation involved. You can't avoid eating so there's really no way around it! There is also the constant emotional burden of needing to be vigilant, watch your child, and check everything they eat. This book will support you through this process.

Beyond this, there are other key times in life where food allergies can become a major issue. Introducing solid foods to babies with known allergies can be worrisome, so I've included the latest research-based advice on how best to do this. Finding childcare or starting school can be tough, because you have to put your trust in others to look after your child and keep them safe. At some point in your allergy journey, you may be advised to try reintroducing the food your child was allergic to, to see if they have grown out of their allergy. This can be a time of great uncertainty, and it is difficult to shift your mindset away from total avoidance of the food, to deliberately giving them something that you know could make them feel unwell. If they don't grow out of their allergy, the teenage years will bring more readjustment as you gradually hand over responsibility for managing allergies to your child.

I've also intended this book to be helpful to grandparents, relatives, friends and even childcare providers. Anyone who has an interest in looking after your child or providing food for them. It's not always easy to broach the subject, and people may not understand if they haven't experienced it themselves, so it you may like to ask them to read the relevant chapters of this book.

This book provides general advice and should be helpful no matter what food allergies your child has. This advice should also be relevant if your child has multiple allergies like my daughter. While writing this book I've tried to consider children with severe allergic reactions who require an epipen, those who have milder reactions such as vomiting, diarrhoea or hives, and other types of allergies such as FPIES or EoE.

In parts there is a little more discussion over cow's milk allergy. This is because it is the most common allergy in young children, and because cow's milk usually forms such a large part of a child's diet. In other areas there is more discussion of nut and peanut allergies, as these tend to be more severe and need special consideration.

At the end of each chapter you will find relevant links to websites, blogs, journal articles and videos, so that you can go deeper into a topic if you need to.

One thing I deliberately haven't included in this book is recipes. This is for two reasons. Firstly, everyone's allergies are different and it's impossible to cater for everyone's needs. Secondly, there are many recipes available freely online, including on my own website www.myallergykitchen.com.

My main message to allergy parents is not to let allergies stand in your way. Don't allow food allergies to stop your child from doing anything they want to do. You can always find a way for them to join in safely. You child can still have all the amazing childhood experiences that their peers will have, you just might have to do things a little differently. Keep a positive attitude – you can do it! In addition, growing up with the additional challenge of food allergies will make your child a stronger and more empathic person. In other words, having food allergies will help to shape them into an amazing adult!

OUR STORY

My youngest daughter, Ellie, showed signs of food allergy from the day she was born. In the hospital, she vomited profusely after every breastfeed. I had packed plenty of spare clothes in my hospital bag, but I had to send my husband out to buy more! We were only in hospital for around 12 hours, as she was born at 4.30am and we were home by dinnertime the next day.

Once we got home she developed further symptoms. She cried excessively – up to 6 hours a day. She would draw her knees up in pain. She would strain and struggle to pass wind or poo. And she was still bringing up a lot of milk after every feed. Luckily a breastfeeding peer supporter told me about a study that had shown that colic improves when the mother cuts dairy from her diet. So, with Ellie at the grand old age of 2 weeks, I went dairy free.

Within a few days we had seen a massive improvement in Ellie's symptoms. After 2 weeks on a dairy exclusion diet, I had a dairy-fest for a day to see what would happen. All of the symptoms she had before came flooding back, along with a very unpleasant rash of eczema all over her face. It was very clear that dairy was a problem for her. I spoke to a health visitor and she told me to continue on the dairy free diet – but there was no mention of a referral for allergy testing or even to see a dietitian for support.

Naturally, as I went dairy free I began to eat and drink more foods containing soya. I started drinking soya lattes and I began to notice that Ellie seemed to be suffering the day after I had had one. So, I stopped drinking soya milk, and the symptoms went away again. However, I wasn't strict about avoiding foods containing small amounts of soya.

Then, at around 4 months old, Ellie developed what I thought was a tummy bug. She suddenly started filling her nappy with nasty green poos about 14 times a day. She still wasn't better after a week, so I went to the doctor. He said it was nothing to worry about as she wasn't dehydrated, and to give it more time to get better. A few days later she developed a temperature as well, so back to the doctor I went. He referred me to a paediatrician at our local hospital the same day. They diagnosed gastroenteritis and sent us home again.

However, 2 weeks later she still wasn't better. Her temperature had gone back to normal, but she was still doing green poos several times through the day and night, as well as waking frequently and crying in the night. We went back to the GP and saw a different doctor this time, who said she was just a naughty baby. His advice? Leave her to cry. I asked about the green poos and he just completely dismissed me, saying that there is a wide range of 'normal' for babies' poo. I asked if it could be another food allergy, bearing in mind we already knew she was allergic to milk. He suggested 'Oh yes, you could try cutting out some things' and sent me on my way.

I felt so utterly confused about what to do. My gut instinct was that soya was causing these problems. I already knew that soya milk made Ellie feel unwell, so I decided to do another exclusion diet and avoid all forms of soya in all foods and see what would happen. Thankfully this resolved the problem immediately. I did find it incredibly difficult though, as I discovered that soya lecithin is in so many foods – especially the ones that are dairy free!

At around 6 months of age, we started weaning. I didn't get the memo that for children with allergies, it's best to introduce one new food at a time, particularly for those foods that commonly cause allergic reactions. We just went for it. We did baby-led weaning, including Ellie in our family meals, and giving her the same as we were eating.

I did notice that she was more unsettled after we started giving her solid foods. However I just put this down to her body getting used to digesting solids. Then I thought maybe it was a developmental spurt, or teething, or a cold… I was never really quite sure what was going on.

By the time she was 10 months old, Ellie was still waking up to 10 times a night. Several times a week, she would cry for 2-3 hours in the middle of the night, and the only thing that would settle her was to pace up and down with her in my arms. During the day, she would only nap in the sling. If I tried to put her down for a nap, she would fall asleep and then wake up screaming after 10 minutes. I used to joke that she needed more attention when she was asleep than when she was awake. At one point I was so sleep deprived that I started hallucinating. After one particularly bad night we went to see the out of hours doctor, who was utterly baffled and couldn't find anything wrong with her. He just shrugged his shoulders and said 'It's a mystery.'

Ellie would also scream in her car seat, so much so that I stopped driving anywhere by myself unless it was absolutely essential because I found it so distressing. I would end up in tears myself! On family outings at the weekend, my husband would drive and I would sit in the back with Ellie and sing to her to try and calm her down. I think the position of the car seat was squashing her already sore stomach and making her feel even more uncomfortable.

At the same time, Ellie also developed a few small patches of mild eczema on her arms and torso. Her older sister has eczema too, so we recognised it straight away. We started applying moisturizing creams to soothe her dry, itchy skin.

Looking back, it was one of the most stressful times of my life. Every day was just about getting through the day, and life became about doing whatever it took to get a bit more sleep. I felt bad that I wasn't getting to enjoy the time with my baby. I felt like a rubbish mum because I was too tired to do anything with my older daughter. Because of the lack of support from the doctors we had seen, I thought that I was going crazy to think that there was anything wrong, or else just a bad mum who didn't know how to look after my baby.

Eventually I began to realise that this was a problem that wasn't going to go away on its own. I went back to the doctors and saw a different GP again this time. I explained that I had been researching Ellie's symptoms online and thought that she might have reflux. He prescribed baby Gaviscon, which we tried for a couple of weeks with no improvement. I started to keep a food and symptoms diary and noticed that the 'bad nights' always came after I had eaten certain foods. I went back and suggested that it could be more allergies. The doctor agreed with me that we should both do yet another exclusion diet (as I was still breastfeeding). It was really tough as I had to cut out gluten, oats, eggs and legumes, in addition to milk and soya. We basically ate a very healthy caveman-style diet of meat, fish, vegetables, fruit, potatoes, rice, nuts and seeds.

Thankfully all the hard work was worth it as Ellie started to get much better. She started sleeping better, she stopped crying in the night and in her car seat, and her eczema went away. I went back to the doctor who immediately referred me to a paediatrician for allergy testing. It was such a relief to finally have acknowledgement that my instincts had been right, there was a real problem and we really did need some help!

We finally saw the paediatrician when Ellie was 14 months old. He said 'I don't know why you are here, you have already done all the hard work yourself!' He did send Ellie for blood tests, but we didn't have skin prick tests as her reactions were mainly gastrointestinal. The blood tests came back with mildly raised IgE antibodies, but all the individual foods they tested for came back negative. The paediatrician said this just showed that the tests weren't very useful! He diagnosed all of Ellie's allergies based on her symptoms and the results of the exclusion diet.

Getting the diagnosis was such a relief. Ellie had suffered so much in the first year of her life and it was wonderful when she started to feel so much better. I was also relieved that there was such a simple solution to the problem (i.e. don't eat the foods). And, although she still woke up in the night, she just wanted a quick cuddle and then went straight back to sleep. My husband and I finally started to feel a bit more human again, instead of dragging ourselves through every day as sleep deprived zombies.

Now flash forward – at the time of writing Ellie is 4 and a half years old. She has thankfully outgrown some of her allergies and is now only allergic to foods containing uncooked dairy products, and soya in any form. She went to preschool from just before her 3rd birthday, and in September she started at school. For all intents and purposes, she is a happy, healthy, normal child. She gets to join in with everything her friends do, it just takes a bit more organisation to make it happen.

Looking back, I feel so bad that Ellie was basically suffering and in pain for most of the first year of her life. I feel let down that none of the doctors we saw picked up on her food allergies until she was a year old, despite the fact we already knew she was an allergic person. I also feel guilty because before I had Ellie, I did used to think that people with food allergies were just complaining over a bit of stomach ache. Now I know the reality of it! And my mission with this book is to help others going through the same thing.

Thank you for reading!

CHAPTER 1

DOES MY CHILD HAVE A FOOD ALLERGY?

WHAT ARE FOOD ALLERGIES AND INTOLERANCES?

Although people often mix up the terms 'food allergy' and 'food intolerance', they actually mean different things. True food allergies are caused by the immune system reacting to a food as if it is something harmful. Food intolerances do not involve the immune system and problems are caused when the body cannot digest the food properly. This book focuses only on food allergies.

Food allergies are more common in children than adults. This is because children often outgrow their allergies, usually before the age of five. In the UK, it is currently estimated that between one and two percent of adults and five to eight percent of children suffer from food allergies. This is equivalent to around two million people in total. It represents around two children in every school classroom. A small proportion (less than ten percent) of these will be at risk of anaphylaxis, a severe, life-threatening reaction.

The number of babies born with food allergies has increased rapidly in recent decades. UK hospital admissions for food allergies have risen by seven times since 1990. The reason for this is not yet known, although scientists are trying to find out why. Multiple food allergies are also becoming more commonplace, and about thirty percent of children with food allergies are allergic to more than one type of food.

Allergies tend to run in families, and are often linked with asthma, eczema and hayfever. Together, these conditions are known as 'atopy'. Food allergies are more likely to develop if the child already has asthma, eczema or hayfever, or if parents or siblings have ever had food allergies, asthma, eczema or hayfever.

Allergic reactions to food can happen immediately or be delayed by several hours or even days. Severe allergic reactions are rare, but can be fatal and require urgent medical attention. In the UK, around 10 people die each year from such allergic reactions. Mild allergic reactions are less dramatic but can still be uncomfortable and worrying. Immediate reactions are known as IgE-mediated allergies and delayed reactions are known as non-IgE-mediated allergies. People sometimes have a mixture of both types.

IgE-mediated allergies are caused by the body producing an antibody called Immunoglobulin E (or IgE for short) either shortly after or within a few hours of eating the food allergen, or sometimes just by touching the food. This antibody tells the body that it is being attacked by a foreign invader, and that it needs to release a substance called histamine to get rid of the allergen. This can cause unpleasant symptoms affecting the whole body. These are sometimes called immediate reactions because they usually happen within two hours of eating the food.

Non-IgE-mediated allergies are caused by a different type of immune response, which doesn't affect the whole body. They are sometimes known as cell-mediated allergies. These type of reactions are usually more delayed and may appear after 2 hours and within 3 days of eating the food. Symptoms typically affect mainly the digestive system. Non-IgE allergies can also be associated with eczema.

There is currently no cure for food allergies. To prevent a reaction, people with food allergies must strictly avoid the food they are allergic to. Mild IgE-mediated reactions can be treated with antihistamines. Severe IgE-mediated reactions are treated with epinephrine, which is prescribed in the form of an auto-injector such as an Epi-Pen, Jext or Emerade. There is no treatment for non-IgE reactions.

People can be allergic to any food, but the most common allergens are peanuts, tree nuts, egg, milk, wheat, fish, soya and sesame. People with allergies can have different levels of sensitivity. For example, many people with egg allergy can eat baked egg (e.g. in cakes) with no problems. For very sensitive individuals, an allergic reaction can occur to tiny amounts of the food and in extremely rare cases can even be caused by skin contact with the food or food particles in the air.

COELIAC DISEASE

Coeliac disease is not a food allergy. It is an immune response to gluten, which is found in grains such as wheat, barley and rye. If a person with coeliac disease eats gluten, their immune system attacks the lining of the small intestine. They may experience unpleasant symptoms such as bloating, diarrhoea, vomiting, stomach pains, nausea, wind, constipation, sudden or unexpected weight loss, tiredness, mouth ulcers, anaemia and hair loss. It is known as an autoimmune disease, as the body attacks itself.

If you think your child may be allergic to wheat, it is important to rule out coeliac disease first. This is a lifelong condition which affects around 1 in 100 people. If left untreated, coeliac disease can lead to nutritional deficiencies and other complications.

SIGNS AND SYMPTOMS OF POSSIBLE FOOD ALLERGY

The next few pages explain the symptoms of different types of food allergy, including immediate and delayed reactions, FPIES, FPIAP, EO and symptoms to look for in babies. Food allergies can affect different areas of the body, including the skin, respiratory system, and digestive system. Your child may not have all the symptoms listed. Allergic reactions can also be different every time. The next chapter will explain how to keep track of your child's symptoms to help you and your healthcare professional to reach a diagnosis.

SYMPTOMS OF IGE-MEDIATED FOOD ALLERGY
(Immediate reactions: within 2 hours of eating the food)

Feeling lightheaded or faint
Difficulty swallowing or
speaking
Confusion and anxiety
Collapsing or losing
consciousness
Becoming weak and floppy

Swelling under the skin,
especially lips, face and
around the eyes
Swelling of the lips,
tongue and palate.
Itchy mouth
Itchy nose
Runny nose
Sneezing
Congestion

Feeling sick
Stomach pain
Being sick
Diarrhoea

Breathing difficulties
Wheezing
Clammy skin
Changes in heart rate
Drop in blood pressure
Coughing
Chest tightness
Wheezing
Shortness of breath

Red and/or itchy skin
Red, raised, bumpy, itchy
rash (hives)
(Can appear anywhere on
the body)

© iStock.com/Mashot

SYMPTOMS OF NON-IGE-MEDIATED FOOD ALLERGY
(Delayed reactions: 2 hours – 3 days after eating the food)

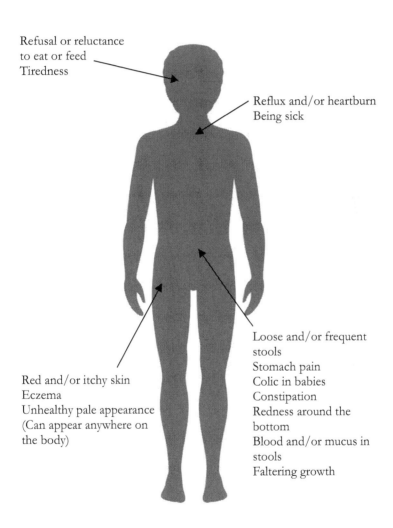

Refusal or reluctance
to eat or feed
Tiredness

Reflux and/or heartburn
Being sick

Red and/or itchy skin
Eczema
Unhealthy pale appearance
(Can appear anywhere on
the body)

Loose and/or frequent
stools
Stomach pain
Colic in babies
Constipation
Redness around the
bottom
Blood and/or mucus in
stools
Faltering growth

© iStock.com/Mashot

ANAPHYLAXIS

Anaphylaxis, or anaphylactic shock, is a severe allergic reaction which can be life-threatening. Anaphylactic reactions usually happen within seconds or minutes of eating the food. They can also happen immediately on skin contact with the food (without it being eaten) and in very rare cases can be airborne. These type of reactions come on very suddenly and can get worse very quickly.

Please note: Anaphylaxis is a medical emergency which needs immediate medical treatment. If you suspect your child is having an anaphylactic reaction dial 999 and ask for an ambulance.

FPIES

Food Protein-Induced Enterocolitis Syndrome (FPIES) is a severe type of delayed food allergy, which is most common in babies and young children. It can cause profuse vomiting within thirty to sixty minutes of feeding, after which the baby may become very drowsy and sleepy. Sometimes babies can develop low blood pressure, or even go into shock, which needs hospital treatment. Fortunately, most children outgrow this type of allergy by the age of five. However, some children with FPIES will go on to develop immediate food allergies.

FPIAP

Food Protein-Induced Allergic Proctocolitis (FPIAP) is a harmless condition of bloody stools in a baby that seems otherwise well. Symptoms usually start within the first month of life. It is usually outgrown by twelve months of age.

EOSINOPHILIC OESOPHAGITIS (EO OR EOE)

The oesophagus is the tube which connects the mouth to the stomach. In EO, the lining of the oesophagus fills with white blood cells and becomes inflamed. This can be caused by an immune reaction to certain foods. The condition may be treated by changing the diet and/or with steroids.

Children with EO may have symptoms similar to reflux, such as vomiting, discomfort and pain. As a result, children with EO may refuse to eat and fail to gain weight. It is more common in boys and men. It is often associated with eczema and asthma.

EO is diagnosed by putting a camera down the throat so the doctor can see inside your child's oesophagus. A small tissue sample (biopsy) will also be taken from the lining of the oesophagus at the same time. Your child may need blood tests and/or skin prick tests to identify which foods are causing the inflammation – see Chapter 2 for more details of these.

SYMPTOMS OF FOOD ALLERGY IN BABIES

It can be particularly difficult to diagnose food allergies in babies, as they cannot tell us how they are feeling. Here are some possible signs to look for:

- Excessive crying and fussiness – also known as colic.
- Excessive wind or trapped wind – babies may draw their knees up in pain, or strain to pass wind.
- Constipation – in breastfed babies their poo may still be runny, but they may seem to find it hard to pass their poo. Again, they may be pulling their knees up or straining.
- Diarrhoea – this is hard to spot in a breastfed baby as their poo is usually runny anyway, but if they are filling their nappy very frequently it may be classed as diarrhoea. Poos may also be 'explosive', requiring a change of clothes.
- Green poo – green poo can be caused by milk passing through the body too quickly and not being fully digested.
- Mucousy/bloody poo – mucus or blood may be present in the poo due to the body's immune response trying to fight against the allergens in their milk.
- Reflux/vomiting – it is normal for babies to bring up a small amount of milk after a feed but if they are often bringing up larger amounts or even a whole feed this is not normal. In extreme cases babies may projectile vomit.

- Eczema/skin rashes/nappy rash
- Frequent feeding or overfeeding - breastfed babies feed for comfort as well as hunger. If they have stomach ache and feel uncomfortable they may feed more often than usual. In some cases, this can also lead to excessive weight gain.
- Refusing feeds - confusingly, this can also be a symptom if baby associates feeding with pain and discomfort. In this case baby may be slow to gain weight.
- Nasal congestion or cold-like symptoms
- Allergic conjunctivitis – red, itchy, watery eyes
- Difficulty sleeping – babies may have difficulty settling to sleep, or may only be able to sleep in a caregiver's arms, in a sling, or in a reclined position such as a car seat or pushchair. They may also wake excessively and struggle to settle back to sleep.

OTHER SYMPTOMS

Other physical symptoms are also possible in addition to those listed above, but this is rare. Some people believe that a range of mental, behavioural and emotional symptoms could be triggered by food allergies. There is a higher than usual rate of food allergies in children on the autism spectrum, for example – about 36% of children with ASD also have food allergies. However, although a link has been found, it is not certain that one could cause the other. There are many stories online of parents who claim to have improved their child's behaviour or mood simply by changing their diet. However, there is little scientific evidence to back this up at the moment, and so doctors will not usually diagnose food allergies based on this alone.

WHAT TO DO IF YOU SUSPECT A FOOD ALLERGY

You should speak to your GP if you think your child has a food allergy. Make a note of the symptoms your child is having, and when they happen. Take photos of symptoms like skin rashes or even the contents of nappies. If you think you know which food(s) your child is reacting to, tell your doctor. When you speak to your doctor make sure to describe the worst type of reaction – now is not the time to put on a brave face. Your doctor may refer you to an allergy clinic or paediatrician for allergy testing or to a dietitian for help with an exclusion diet and nutritional advice, depending on how severe your child's reactions are and whether you already know what is causing the allergic reactions. There are other conditions that your doctor may wish to rule out first, such as coeliac disease (an illness which is caused by gluten, which is found in wheat and other cereals). You can find out more about allergy tests and exclusion diets in the next chapter.

Getting a diagnosis for food allergies is not easy and can take a long time. The symptoms overlap with a number of other conditions. Very few GPs have had any allergy training and so they may not recognise the signs. You may need to refer them to the iMAP Guideline for Cow's Milk Allergy and the NICE Guideline CG116 for food allergy in children (links at the end of this chapter). Read on to Chapter 2 for more about getting a diagnosis.

KEY POINTS

- Food allergies are an immune system response to a food protein.
- Allergic reactions can be immediate or delayed.
- IgE-mediated allergic reactions happen within two hours of eating the food.
- Non-IgE-mediated allergic reactions happen after two hours of eating the food and within seventy two hours.
- If you suspect your child has a food allergy, speak to your GP for advice.

REFERENCES AND LINKS

- Allergy UK, 'iMAP Guideline' (December 2016), https://www.allergyuk.org/health-professionals/mapguideline, accessed 5th December 2018.
- Allergy UK, 'Types of Food Allergy', https://www.allergyuk.org/information-and-advice/conditions-and-symptoms/36-food-allergy, accessed 5th December 2018.

- Cassels, Tracy, 'Elimination Diets: Food Sensitivities in the Breastfed Baby', *Evolutionary Parenting* [blog] (2015), http://evolutionaryparenting.com/elimination-diets-food-sensitivities-in-the-breastfed-baby/, accessed 5th December 2018.

- Children's Hospital of Philadelphia, 'IgE-Mediated Food Allergies' (January 2014), http://www.chop.edu/conditions-diseases/ige-mediated-food-allergies, accessed 5th December 2018.

- CMPA Support, 'Symptoms', https://cowsmilkproteinallergysupport.webs.com/sympto ms, accessed 5th December 2018.

- Fox, Adam, 'Cow's Milk Allergy Frequently Asked Questions', *Nutrimagen Healthcare Professional*, http://hcp.nutramigen.co.uk/files/6613/4978/0162/CM A_FAQs.pdf, accessed 5th December 2018.

- FPIES UK https://www.fpiesuk.org/, accessed 5th December 2018.

- Holgate, Stephen T and Ewan, Pamela W, 'Allergy: the unmet need', *Royal College of Physicians* (June 2003), https://www.bsaci.org/pdf/allergy_the_unmet_need.pdf, accessed 5th December 2018.

- KellyMom, 'Dairy and other Food Sensitives in Breastfed Babies' (January 2018), http://kellymom.com/health/baby-health/food-sensitivity/, accessed 5th December 2018.

- Knott, Laurence, 'Eosinophilic Oesophagitis', *Patient* (September 2016), https://patient.info/health/dyspepsia-indigestion/eosinophilic-oesophagitis, accessed 5th December 2018.

- National Institute for Health and Clinical Excellence, 'Food allergy in under 19s: assessment and diagnosis', *NICE Guideline CG116* (February 2011), https://www.nice.org.uk/guidance/cg116/, accessed 5th December 2018.

- Nowak-Wegrzyn, Anna, 'Food protein-induced enterocolitis syndrome and allergic proctocolitis', *Allergy and Asthma Proceedings*, 36/3 (2015) 172-84 doi: 10.2500/aap.2015.36.3811

CHAPTER 2

GETTING A DIAGNOSIS

Does your child have some of the symptoms described in Chapter 1? The next step is to work out if food allergies are the cause, and which food(s) they are allergic to. This may be easier said than done. Immediate reactions are easier to pick up on. But if your child has delayed reactions, it may take some detective work to figure out the trigger food(s).

TESTING

The NHS currently uses 2 types of tests to diagnose food allergies: skin prick tests and blood tests. These can only be used to diagnose IgE-mediated allergies (immediate reactions). Doctors can also repeat these tests as your child grows up, to find out whether they have grown out of their allergies or not. Non-IgE-mediated allergies (delayed reactions) are diagnosed by an exclusion diet, which is explained in full detail later in this chapter.

Skin prick tests

A drop containing a small amount of the food is placed on the skin, usually on the forearm. The skin is then pricked through the food droplet. This can be done for several different types of food at once. Two additional pricks are made to check the test has worked properly. The first is done with a drop of saline (salt water) for a definite negative result. The second is done with histamine (the substance that causes immediate allergic reactions) for a definite positive result. After 15-20 minutes the doctor will look at the skin. A large red raised spot (at least 3mm) shows a positive reaction, meaning your child is allergic to that food.

Skin tests are not always completely accurate. A negative reaction is more accurate than a positive one. This means, if your child has a negative reaction, you can be confident in ruling out an allergy to that food. However, if your child has a positive reaction, this may or may not mean your child is allergic to that food. Your doctor will advise you how to interpret your child's test results. Your doctor will likely recommend that your child avoids the food to be on the safe side, until the tests can be repeated when they are older.

The advantage of this test is you get the results very quickly. However, there is a very small risk of anaphylaxis with a skin prick test, so these should only be carried out where resuscitation facilities are available such as an allergy clinic, hospital or larger GP surgery. If you are having tests done privately, make sure these facilities are available.

Blood tests

These are sometimes called RAST tests. A sample of blood is taken and tested for the presence of IgE antibodies. A high level of IgE antibodies may mean that your child has an allergy. There can be other causes, so a doctor must interpret the results. They can also be used to screen for individual food allergies. However, they do not always pick up every food allergy, so it is possible to get a negative test result and still be highly allergic to a food. Some foods contain a large number of different allergens and the test cannot pick up all of them. The test is completely safe, but you do have to wait a few days for the results.

Blood tests can also be used to rule out other potential causes of your child's symptoms, such as coeliac disease (an autoimmune reaction to wheat). If you suspect that wheat is a problem, you must do this before you take it out of your child's diet, otherwise the test will not work. You can only test for coeliac disease if you are eating wheat as a regular part of your diet, more than once a day, for at least six weeks before having the test.

Other types of test

Other tests are available to buy privately but they do not give accurate results. They can be bought online, in health food shops and from alternative health practitioners. A doctor would not use these types of tests to confirm a food allergy. If you are tempted to try any of these tests, don't waste your money!

- Vega test – uses a machine to detect changes in your 'energy levels' in response to different foods.
- Applied Kinesiology – claims to detect allergies based on muscle weakness in response to different foods.
- Hair analysis – claims to detect food allergies by testing a sample of hair.
- IgG blood tests – these test the blood for IgG antibodies, however there is no evidence that these antibodies are linked to food allergies.

EXCLUSION DIET

Non-IgE-mediated (delayed) food allergies can only be diagnosed by an exclusion diet. This means cutting out any foods you think your child may be reacting to for a few weeks to see if symptoms improve. Then, you will reintroduce the food(s) one at a time to see if the symptoms return, and see which food(s) cause a problem.

If you are exclusively breastfeeding and you think your baby has a non-IgE food allergy, you will need to cut the food(s) out of your own diet. If your baby is already weaning, or for an older child, you will need to cut the food(s) out of their diet. Some foods are easier to cut out than others. You may want to speak to a dietitian for detailed advice on which foods to avoid and what you can eat instead, and whether you/your child needs to take supplements to avoid nutritional deficiencies.

An exclusion diet can also be done at home, and will provide you with evidence if you are struggling to get your doctor or healthcare provider to listen to you. Sadly, not all doctors are clued up about food allergies and you may need to be persistent to get a diagnosis.

Step 1: Keep a food diary

Keeping a food diary is a way to make a shortlist of foods you think your child may be reacting to. If you already know which food(s) you think your child is reacting to, you can skip this step and go straight onto step 2. In the UK, the most common food allergies in babies and children are milk, egg, peanuts, tree nuts, fish and shellfish. Wheat, gluten, soy, sesame and kiwi can also commonly cause problems, but it is possible to be allergic to any type of food. If anyone else in the family already has food allergies, these foods are potential suspects too.

To keep a food diary, write down in as much detail as you can everything your child eats and drinks including all food and drink, medicines, supplements, snacks, sweets and even licking the bowl when cooking together. For babies who are breastfeeding you need to write down everything you eat as well, along with your baby's symptoms. Do this for two weeks, continuing to eat as normal, without making any changes to your child's diet.

Make a note if your child is teething or has a cold or other illness. Keep food packaging so that you and your health professional can check ingredients.

On the next page you will find an example of a completed food diary. You can download your own blank template to use from my own website at www.myallergykitchen.com/downloads or alternatively use an app such as AlliApp or MySymptoms.

Once you have completed the food diary you should speak to a doctor or dietitian and see if you can work out which food(s) might be causing a problem. Then you can go on to the next stage and get ready to cut the suspect allergen(s) out of your child's diet (and/or your own, if you are breastfeeding).

Example food diary

Date	Time	Food eaten	Symptoms
7th March	5.30 am	Milk feed	Woke early with tummy ache, wind and diarrhoea. Did 3 loose, mucousy poos in 30 minutes.
	7 am	Scrambled eggs, bacon, baked beans	
	9.30 am	Milk feed	
	10 am	Banana and rice cakes	
	12 noon	Spaghetti & meatballs with tomato sauce and grated cheese on top Yogurt	Clingy and whiny during the afternoon.
	1 pm	Milk feed	
	4 pm	Breadsticks & houmous	
	6 pm	Roast chicken breast, roast potatoes, carrots, peas, broccoli and gravy Chocolate cake & custard	Rash on face after eating pudding.
	7 pm	Milk feed	Tummy looked bloated.
	2 am	Milk feed	Awake and crying for an hour. Wouldn't resettle even after feeding.

Step 2: Prepare

Go through your cupboards and check ingredients. Think about what products you need to replace and what alternatives you will use instead. If you are cutting out dairy, do not switch straight to soya as it is not unusual to be allergic to both. Use almond, coconut or hemp milk instead. Rice milk is not suitable for children under 5 years old, because it contains tiny amounts of arsenic!

'Free From' products tend to be expensive, very processed and not always particularly healthy, but it may help to buy a few treats, or basics like bread, while you complete the exclusion diet. This can help to make the transition easier, so you don't/your child doesn't feel too deprived. You may also like to make a meal plan to make life easier – there is more on how to do this in Chapter 5. Make sure your fridge and cupboards are stocked with plenty of things your child can eat.

For support you can speak to a dietitian, and there are lots of allergy groups on Facebook for cow's milk protein allergy (CMPA), gluten-free diets, coeliac disease etc where you can find recipe ideas, restaurant reviews and lists of safe foods, as well as asking questions or advice.

Step 3: Eliminate food(s) from your child's diet

Stop your child from eating all of the foods you think might be causing a problem. This might only be one or two foods, or it could be several foods. It is harder to cut out lots of different allergens at once, but you will see results faster than cutting them out one at a time. If your child does have multiple food allergies, they won't feel completely better until all problem foods are eliminated. It may seem overwhelming at first, but you will soon learn what your child can eat safely.

Dairy may take around 2 weeks to get out of your child's system, gluten can take 6 weeks. See if you notice any improvement in symptoms during this time. Make sure you check the packets of everything your child eats and check before eating out. Most chain restaurants have allergen information available online. All restaurants are required by law to provide information on any of the 14 most common allergens used as ingredients in their food so it is still possible to eat out safely – just ask. See Chapter 6 for more help with eating out.

You might find that your child's symptoms get worse during the exclusion diet. This could mean that they are allergic to another food that they are eating more of whilst on the exclusion diet. For example, if you switch from dairy to coconut milk and their symptoms worsen, this may mean that coconut is a problem for them. Make a note of it and try a different alternative.

Step 4: Evaluate and Reintroduce

If you have seen a noticeable improvement in symptoms over the 6-week period, then an allergy or intolerance is the most likely cause. Try reintroducing each eliminated food, one at a time, to see if symptoms come back. Start with a small amount of the food and gradually increase. Do this over a few days and then wait three days before reintroducing any other foods, to allow time for any delayed symptoms to appear. If the symptoms do not come back then it is safe to include that food in your child's diet again. If they do come back then this confirms the allergy and you should discuss this with your doctor or dietitian. They will help you decide whether to avoid the food completely, or whether your child can tolerate a small amount. For example, some children with egg allergy can tolerate baked egg.

FORMULA FEEDING AND COW'S MILK ALLERGY

If your baby is formula fed and you think they are allergic to cow's milk, speak to your doctor about trying alternative milks. You may need to try a few different types of milk until your baby settles, or combine one of the milks with medication to control symptoms.

There are two types of formula which are suitable for babies with cow's milk allergy. They are both known as 'hypoallergenic' formula, meaning less likely to cause a reaction, and are only available on prescription. **Extensively hydrolysed formula**

(EHF) is made from cow's milk where the proteins are broken down to prevent a reaction, and is tolerated in most babies with mild to moderate non-IgE cow's milk allergy. If your baby still doesn't settle on this type of formula, your doctor can also prescribe **amino acid formula** (AAF). This contains no cow's milk protein and is suitable for the most sensitive babies. It is still nutritionally complete. You may need to try more than one brand of formula before you find one that suits your baby. You can also use these formulas in cooking once your baby starts weaning.

In the shops you can buy formula made from the milk of other mammals such as goats, sheep, etc. which do not contain cow's milk protein. However, the proteins in goat/sheep milk are very similar to cow's milk and there is a high chance that your child will still react to them. For this reason, you should not give them to babies with cow's milk allergy unless advised by a doctor.

Soya formula may be suggested for babies over six months if EHF and AAF are not tolerated, as long as there is no soya allergy. However, its use is controversial for a number of reasons. Firstly, soya contains a substance which is similar to the human hormone oestrogen. This may affect babies as they grow, as their development is sensitive to oestrogens. As young babies only drink milk, they would take in a much higher proportion of these substances than children or adults who eat or drink soya as part of a varied diet. This has not been proven, but some parents prefer to avoid soya as a precaution. Secondly, soya formula contains a type of sugar called glucose, which is more harmful to your baby's teeth than normal milk sugars. Therefore, you should only use soya formula if it has been recommended by a medical professional.

Other types of formula that are not suitable for babies with cow's milk allergies are lactose-free formula and partially hydrolysed formula or 'comfort milk'. These are still made from cow's milk and will still cause an allergic reaction.

DIAGNOSIS

Food allergies can either be diagnosed by tests or by an exclusion diet. This can be a stressful process for both you and your child.

You may have mixed feelings about your child's diagnosis. If it comes after a sudden severe reaction, it may be quite a traumatic experience. You may need some time to come to terms with what has happened (see Chapter 15). However if you have had a long wait for diagnosis, it may be a relief to finally have some answers to your questions.

KEY POINTS

- The two main tests doctors use to diagnose food allergies are skin prick tests and blood tests.
- Other types of tests are unreliable.
- Sometimes doctors will recommend doing an exclusion diet to diagnose food allergies.
- Keeping a food diary can help to identify which food(s) your child may be reacting to.
- Formula fed babies with suspected cow's milk allergy can try special hypoallergenic formula, available on prescription.

REFERENCES AND LINKS

- Allergy UK, 'iMAP Guideline' (December 2016), https://www.allergyuk.org/health-professionals/mapguideline, accessed 5th December 2018.
- Coeliac UK 'Blood Tests' https://www.coeliac.org.uk/coeliac-disease/getting-diagnosed/blood-tests/ , accessed 5th December 2018.
- Gavura, Scott, 'IgG Food Intolerance Tests: What does the science say?', *Science-Based Medicine* [blog] (February 2012), https://sciencebasedmedicine.org/igg-food-intolerance-tests-what-does-the-science-say/, accessed 5th December 2018.
- Morris, Adrian, 'Allergy Testing', *Surrey Allergy Clinic* (November 2016), https://www.allergy-clinic.co.uk/our-clinics/allergy-testing/, accessed 5th December 2018.
- Nanny Care, 'Why goat milk?' (2014), http://www.nannycare.co.uk/why-goat-milk/, accessed 5th December 2018.

- NHS, 'Food Allergy: Diagnosis' (May 2016), https://www.nhs.uk/conditions/food-allergy/diagnosis/, accessed 5th December 2018.
- NHS, 'Types of formula milk' (October 2016), https://www.nhs.uk/Conditions/pregnancy-and-baby/Pages/types-of-infant-formula.aspx, accessed 5th December 2018.

CHAPTER 3

BREASTFEEDING AND WEANING

How to feed your baby is a very personal decision. Everyone's circumstances are different, and you have to make the best choice to suit your family situation. This chapter covers information on breastfeeding and weaning to help you make an informed decision about how you want to feed your child. Your health professional can make specific recommendations for your child's individual needs. For information on hypoallergenic baby formulas for babies with cow's milk allergy, see Chapter 2.

BREASTFEEDING

For all babies, the NHS recommends exclusive breastfeeding for the first 6 months, and then continuing to breastfeed alongside solid foods for as long as you and your baby want. The World Health Organisation recommends continuing breastfeeding until at least 2 years of age. Breastfeeding provides health benefits for both you and your baby. It is also free and available whenever your baby needs it. In the UK, breastfeeding is very popular and 73% of mothers start off breastfeeding.

Breastfeeding is especially important for babies who already have food allergies, or are at high risk of allergies (if they already have eczema, or asthma, or if there is a history of allergies in the family).

This is because breastfeeding can help to reduce the risk of a baby developing allergies later in life. It may also help to reduce the severity of food allergies in babies who already have them. This is because breastmilk contains substances that help the immune system to develop normally, which are not found in formula milk. Breastfeeding for at least 2 years is the best recommendation for most babies with or at risk of allergies.

Breastfeeding mothers can usually eat whatever they like without any problems. However, what you eat does affect the content of your breastmilk and some babies can show signs of an allergic reaction to what you have eaten. Proteins from the food eaten go into your breastmilk within a few hours. Food allergies in exclusively breastfed babies affects only 1 in 200 babies and is most often caused by cow's milk allergy.

How bad your baby's reactions are will depend on how sensitive they are and how much of the food you have eaten. If your baby is showing signs of allergic reaction most of the time, it may be down to a food that you eat regularly.

ALLERGENS IN BREASTMILK

If your baby has very severe reactions to food allergens via your breastmilk, then your baby's doctor may advise you to stop breastfeeding immediately and switch to hypoallergenic formula. This is because doctors are taught that allergens can stay in breastmilk for up to two weeks. It can be very difficult to switch from breastfeeding to formula and then back again after this amount of time.

But is this really true? Do you have to permanently stop breastfeeding? Some small studies have shown that the amount of food protein in breastmilk peaks just a few hours after eating the food, and then decreases rapidly. Breastmilk may in fact be clear of food allergens in just a day or two. You may only need to use hypoallergenic formula for just 48 hours before returning to breastfeeding, which is much more manageable. If your baby has severe reactions and you would like to continue breastfeeding, you may wish to discuss this research with your doctor.

Note that it may still take up to two weeks for your baby to show signs of improvement, whether you continue to breastfeed or decide to use hypoallergenic formula instead. This is just the time needed for the body to heal.

STUDIES : BREASTMILK AND ALLERGENS

- Vadas, Peter, et al. "Detection of peanut allergens in breast milk of lactating women." *Jama* 285.13 (2001): 1746-1748.
- Palmer, D. J., M. S. Gold, and M. Makrides. "Effect of maternal egg consumption on breast milk ovalbumin concentration." *Clinical & Experimental Allergy* 38.7 (2008): 1186-1191.
- Kilshaw, Peter J., and Andrew J. Cant. "The passage of maternal dietary proteins into human breast milk." *International Archives of Allergy and Immunology* 75.1 (1984): 8-15.
- Troncone, R., et al. "Passage of Gliadin Into Human Breast Milk." *Pediatric Research* 20.7 (1986): 696.
- Chirdo, F. G., et al. "Presence of high levels of non-degraded gliadin in breast milk from healthy mothers." *Scandinavian journal of gastroenterology* 33.11 (1998): 1186-1192.
- Nowak-Węgrzyn A. "Food protein-induced enterocolitis syndrome and allergic proctocolitis." *Allergy and Asthma proceedings* 36.3 (2015): 172-184.

If your baby has mild to moderate reactions you can continue breastfeeding if you want to. If your baby reacts to foods that you have eaten via breastmilk then you will need to stop eating those foods. Your baby may need to have allergy tests to find out what they are allergic to or you may need to do an exclusion diet (see Chapter 2), depending on what your baby's symptoms are.

If your baby does not have allergic reactions to foods you have eaten via breastmilk, you do not need to remove them from your diet and you should continue to eat as normal. Avoiding foods you and your baby are not already allergic to increases the chances of them (or you) developing an allergy.

Chapters 4, 5 and 6 go into more detail about how to avoid food allergens at home and out and about. Although this is not always easy, you will learn a lot about safe foods for your baby. When they start on solid foods themselves, you will need to learn about this anyway. Although it may seem like hard work at first, it is not a reason to stop breastfeeding.

If you have to stop eating particular foods because of your baby's food allergy, you will need to make sure you still have a balanced diet. If your baby is allergic to dairy you will need to take special care to ensure you are getting enough calcium, and if necessary take a calcium supplement. You can ask for a referral to a dietitian who can help you to ensure you are getting all the nutrients you need from your diet.

Breastmilk adapts to meet your baby's needs as they grow and change and will provide all the nutrients they need. This is even more important for a baby with food allergies who will be on a limited diet. Breastmilk also provides a lot of non-nutritional benefits for your baby's immune system.

If your baby is allergic to cow's milk and you are thinking of stopping breastfeeding, remember that your baby will be reliant on special hypoallergenic formula, which is only available on prescription. It can be difficult to get a breastfed baby to drink hypoallergenic formula because it tastes very different. You may also have to try a few different types before you find one that suits your baby.

If you are returning to work it may be easier to express breastmilk for someone else to feed to your baby. Under the law, employers must provide a suitable place for pregnant and breastfeeding mothers to rest and lie down. This does not mean in the toilets! Your employer may also provide you with a fridge to store expressed milk, and allow extra breaks for pumping, but this is not required by law.

Another option is to find childcare close to your work so that you can breastfeed your baby during your breaks. Alternatively, you may decide to continue to breastfeed your baby before and after work, and ask whoever is looking after your child to give them formula milk. If you do decide to switch to formula for any reason, allow plenty of time for your baby to wean onto their new milk before stopping breastfeeding.

GETTING SUPPORT WITH BREASTFEEDING

Breastfeeding, when it is going well, can be a wonderful bonding experience between you and your baby. There are also many health benefits for both mum and baby. However, if it is not going well it can be really hard work and this is when you need to find support. Getting the right help can reassure you that your baby is getting enough milk, that they are growing well, that their fussiness is normal and does not mean that you are a bad mum, and can also point you in the right direction if there is a problem such as tongue tie, or mastitis.

You can get face-to-face support with breastfeeding at a drop-in support group in your local area. Organisations that run groups include SureStart centres, La Leche League, and the National Childbirth Trust (NCT). Groups are often run by 'peer supporters' which means mums who have breastfed at least one baby and who have been on a training course to learn how to help other mums. Plus, you will meet other mums who are at a similar stage to you, who can also be a great source of support.

Peer supporters have been through it all before and can reassure you about what is normal and what is not, providing practical and emotional support. They can check your baby is latching properly and discuss any issues you may be concerned about. If there is a problem they can tell you where to get help in your local area (e.g. where to hire a breast pump, how to get diagnosis of an allergy, or how to get a tongue tie corrected). They can also help you plan how to continue breastfeeding when you return to work.

You can also get face-to-face support from breastfeeding counsellors, who are experienced breastfeeders who have received more in-depth training in providing breastfeeding support. You can find out about local breastfeeding counsellors in your area from drop-in groups, health visitors, midwives, and hospitals.

Lactation consultants are breastfeeding specialists available in some hospitals and privately. They are sometimes referred to as an IBCLC which means 'International Board Certified Lactation Consultant'. This is the highest level of breastfeeding and lactation certification, requiring extensive experience and education. They can provide support in more complex, difficult or high-risk situations. You can find your nearest IBCLC on the Lactation Consultants of Great Britain website at http://www.lcgb.org.

If you can't get to a group for any reason, there are also a number of phonelines you can call for breastfeeding support. Like the drop-in groups these are mainly staffed by peer supporters who volunteer their time to help breastfeeding mums.

Breastfeeding Helplines

NCT Breastfeeding Helpline
0300 330 0700
National Breastfeeding Helpline (government-funded)
0300 100 0212
La Leche League Helpline
0345 120 2918
Association of Breastfeeding Mothers
0300 330 5453

There is also a brilliant online support group on Facebook just for mums who are breastfeeding babies with food allergies, especially cow's milk allergy. It is called CMPA Support for Breastfeeding and can be found at:
https://www.facebook.com/groups/CMPASforBreastFeeding/

WEANING

The current advice from the Department of Health is to introduce solid foods to babies no earlier than 17 weeks and no later than 6 months of age. Babies' digestive systems are not ready for solid foods before 17 weeks. Starting solids before then can actually increase the chances of your baby developing a food allergy.

Ideal first foods are plain fruit and vegetables such as apple, banana, avocado, carrots, butternut squash and sweet potato. All of these foods can be pureed and are sweet tasting. They can also be cut into fingers or sticks to make them easier to pick up for self-feeding. You can also offer starchy foods (such as bread, pasta, potatoes and rice), protein, and pasteurised dairy foods.

Never feed your baby anything you know they are allergic to.

IS MY BABY AT RISK OF FOOD ALLERGY?

Babies who already have a food allergy, or have severe eczema, are at a higher risk of developing further food allergies. You may want to ask for allergy testing before starting weaning, but there can be a long wait for an appointment (which could delay you introducing the foods and actually increase the risk of food allergy). Discuss this with your healthcare professional to decide what is best for your baby.

INTRODUCING ALLERGENIC FOODS

Scientists have found that introducing foods that commonly cause allergies before your baby turns one can actually greatly reduce the chances of them developing an allergy to those foods. You should aim to introduce allergenic foods alongside first foods. This can be done whenever you start weaning, but not before seventeen weeks.

When offering these allergenic foods to your baby, introduce one new food at a time. That way, if they do have a reaction you will know which food has caused the problem. Choose a day when your baby is well. Start with a small amount of the food e.g. half a teaspoon and increase slowly over a few days. Ideally, give them the food in the morning so you can look for signs of a reaction during the day. Don't worry if your baby doesn't eat the food, just try again another day. Once you know they can eat the food without any problems, you can continue to give them the food

Allergenic foods
Milk
Eggs
Wheat
Soya
Fish
Shellfish
Peanuts
Tree nuts
Sesame seeds

regularly (at least once a week). Then you can start to give them another new food.

If they start to show signs of an allergic reaction (see Chapter 1) stop giving the food. If they show signs of an immediate reaction, do not give the food again and speak to your GP. If they show signs of a delayed reaction, the symptoms should get better within a few days. If the symptoms are mild, you can try giving the food again after a week or two. If the symptoms come back after giving the food again, are severe, or your child is not growing, then speak to your GP.

> **If your baby shows signs of a severe reaction dial 999 immediately.**

If someone else in the family already has a food allergy, you need to think about how to feed your baby whilst also keeping the person with the food allergy safe. If you have a food allergy yourself, you may need to ask someone like your partner, relative or friend, to help you do this.

Here are some ideas for introducing allergenic foods. Some companies have started to offer special foods for introducing allergens to babies. These are convenient but not necessary, and it is fine to introduce these allergens using normal family foods. Do not introduce any of these foods if you already know your child is allergic to them:

- Milk
  - Yogurt – look for yogurt with no added sugar or artificial sweeteners, or plain yogurt mixed with fruit puree to sweeten
  - Fromage frais with no added sugar
  - Hard cheese cut into pieces your baby can pick up
  - Soft cheese as a dip or spread
  - Porridge
- Eggs
  - Boiled eggs cut lengthways into fingers
  - Omelette cut into fingers

- Wheat (check ingredients of these products for other allergens)
  - Breadsticks
  - Crackers
  - Pasta
  - Crumpets
  - Rich tea biscuits
  - Homemade bread
  - Be aware that most commercial bread contains soya as well as wheat
- Soya
  - Once you know your child is happy eating wheat, you could give them commercially made bread which contains wheat and soya.
  - Soya yogurt or dessert
- Fish
  - Cod is ideal as it is not too strong tasting. It can be broken into flakes and mixed in with other foods e.g. mashed potato or tomato sauce. It can also be cut into larger pieces for your baby to pick up.
- Shellfish
  - Prawns
  - Crab (note that 'crab sticks' or 'seafood sticks' may contain a mixture of fish and shellfish and should not be given until you already know your child can eat both of these foods)
- Peanuts - Do not give children under 5 whole or chopped peanuts as they are a choking hazard
  - Smooth peanut butter
  - 'Puffed' peanut snacks
  - Peanut powder or peanut flour can be mixed into soft foods such as purees, yogurt etc. or added to milk
- Tree nuts - Do not give children under 5 whole nuts or chopped nuts as they are a choking hazard
  - Nut butters such as almond butter, hazelnut butter, cashew nut butter etc
  - Ground nuts/peanuts can be mixed into soft foods such as purees, yogurt etc. or added to milk

- Sesame seeds
  - Houmous contains sesame and can be given as a dip with vegetable crudités

FREE FROM FOODS

Most 'free from' foods are designed for adults. They are not suitable for babies and young children as they are highly processed and high in sugar and salt. Many foods in the baby aisle will be suitable for babies with allergies such as dried fruit snacks, oaty bars, rice cakes, baby 'crisps' and fruit and vegetable purees. These are convenient when out and about, but not essential. Stick to mainly simple, whole foods as much as possible such as fruit, vegetables, potatoes, rice, pasta, bread, meat, fish, eggs, beans, milk and dairy products (depending on your child's allergies of course).

Remember, you can breastfeed your baby with food allergies for as long as you want to. If you do, take special care to ensure you are getting everything you need from your diet. When you decide to start solids, introduce one new food at a time and introduce allergenic foods early to reduce the risk of more food allergies developing.

KEY POINTS

- You can continue to breastfeed your baby with food allergies for as long as you want to.
- If your baby reacts to food allergens in your breastmilk, you will need to avoid eating the foods they are allergic to.
- You should start to offer your baby solid foods between 17 weeks and 6 months of age.
- Introducing allergenic foods right from the start of weaning may reduce the risk of a food allergy developing.
- Introduce one new food at a time.

REFERENCES AND LINKS

- British Dietetic Association, 'Preventing food allergy in your baby: information for parents' (May 2018)

https://www.bda.uk.com/regionsgroups/groups/foodalle
rgy/resources/infant_feeding_and_allergy_prevention_gui
dance_for_parents, accessed 5th December 2018.

- Du Toit G, Roberts G, Sayre PH, Bahnson HT, Radulovic
S, Santos AF, Brough HA, Phippard D, Basting M, Feeney
M, Turcanu V, Sever ML, et al (2015) Randomized Trial of
Peanut Consumption in Infants at Risk for Peanut Allergy.
The New England Journal of Medicine, 372 (2015), 803-813.
doi: 10.1056/NEJMoa1414850.

- Host, A. and Halken, S., 'Primary prevention of food
allergy in infants who are at risk', *Current Opinion in Allergy
and Clinical Immunology* [abstract], 5, 3, (2005), 255-9. doi:
10.1097/01.all.0000168791.89829.2a

- Infant Nutrition Council, 'Breastmilk Information', (2013)
http://www.infantnutritioncouncil.com/resources/breast
milk-information/, accessed 5th December 2018.

- KellyMom, 'Dairy and other Food Sensitives in Breastfed
Babies' (January 2018),
http://kellymom.com/health/baby-health/food-
sensitivity/, accessed 5th December 2018.

- Lam, Jane, 'Allergies can be beaten with action early in life'
The Standard (2018),
http://www.thestandard.com.hk/section-
news.php?id=192022&sid=4, accessed 5th December 2018.

- Muraro A, Halken S, Arshad SH, Beyer K, Dubois AEJ,
Du Toit G, Eigenmann PA, Grimshaw KEC, Hoest A,
Lack G, O'Mahony L, Papadopoulos NG, Panesar S,
Prescott, Roberts G, de Silva D, Venter C, Verhasselt V,
Akdis AC, Sheikh A, 'EAACI food allergy and anaphylaxis
guidelines. Primary prevention of food allergy' *Allergy*, 69,
5 (2014), 590-601. doi: 10.1111/all.12398.

- NHS, 'Benefits of breastfeeding' (February 2017),
https://www.nhs.uk/conditions/pregnancy-and-
baby/benefits-breastfeeding/, accessed 5th December
2018.

- Paullin, Trillitye, 'True or False: Allergens are Present in
Breast Milk for Weeks', *Free to Feed* [blog] (2018),
https://www.befreetofeed.com/single-post/True-or-
False-Allergens-are-present-in-breast-milk-for-weeks,

accessed 5th December 2018.

- Perkin, M., Kirsty, L., , and Lack, G, 'EAT: Enquiring About Tolerance – A randomized controlled trial of early introduction to allergenic foods to induce tolerance in infants', *Food Standards Agency* (2016), https://www.food.gov.uk/sites/default/files/media/docu ment/eat-study-full-report.pdf , accessed 5th December 2018.

- Roduit C, Frei R, Depner M, Schaub B, Loss G, Genuneit J, Pfefferle P, Hyvärinen A, Karvonen AM, Riedler J, Dalphin JC, Pekkanen J, von Mutius E, Braun-Fahrländer C, Lauener R;, 'Increased food diversity in the first year of life is inversely associated with allergic diseases', *Journal of Allergy and Clinical Immunology*, 133, 4 (2014), 1056–1064 doi: 10.1016/j.jaci.2013.12.1044.

CHAPTER 4

FOOD SHOPPING

Now you know what your child is allergic to, you need to make sure they completely avoid eating the food(s) they react to. If you are breastfeeding then you may also need to avoid their food allergen (see Chapter 3 for more on breastfeeding a baby with food allergies). At the moment this is the only treatment for food allergies, apart from emergency medication such as epi-pens and antihistamines. Giving their immune system a break (from allergic reactions) gives them the best chance of growing out of their allergies.

How strict you need to be depends on your child's tolerance level. For example, some children who are allergic to egg can tolerate baked egg in cakes and biscuits, and some children who are allergic to soya can tolerate soya lecithin, which is found in many processed foods and chocolate. Other individuals can react to even trace amounts in their food, and will need to be much more careful.

This means checking the ingredients of every single item of food you buy, and getting used to cooking with substitute ingredients. Shopping and cooking will take longer and be more expensive, there's no two ways about it. Over time it does get easier as you learn what your child can and can't eat.

READING FOOD LABELS

According to EU law, food allergens have to be labelled in a clear and consistent way whenever they are used as in ingredient in pre-packaged foods. This law came into effect in December 2014 and makes it much easier to make safe food choices. These regulations are set to stay in place after Brexit.

These regulations do not apply to food that is prepared and packed on site, such as independent or in-store bakeries, delicatessens, butchers, fishmongers etc. It also doesn't apply to pre-packed sandwiches, salad etc in cafés, if they are prepared on the premises. The seller must still have the information available if you ask for it, but it doesn't have to be printed on the packaging. This is designed to help small businesses, but also applies to larger companies.

There are 14 allergens which must be emphasised on the label. These are:

- eggs
- milk
- fish
- crustaceans (e.g. crab, lobster, crayfish, shrimp, prawn)
- molluscs (e.g. mussels, oysters, squid)
- peanuts
- tree nuts (namely almonds, hazelnuts, walnuts, cashews, pecans, brazils, pistachios, macadamia nuts or Queensland nuts)
- sesame seeds
- cereals containing gluten (namely wheat (such as spelt, Khorasan wheat/Kamut), rye, barley, oats, or their hybridised strains).
- soya
- celery and celeriac
- mustard
- lupin
- sulphur dioxide and sulphites (at concentration of more than ten parts per million)

Where these foods are used as an ingredient in a pre-packaged food, they may be written in **bold**, *italics*, CAPITALS, highlighted or underlined, to make them stand out. This information must all be in one place. Manufacturers are no longer allowed to put this type of allergen information in a separate box, which means you only need to look at the ingredients section on the packaging. Here are some examples:

INGREDIENTS: Maize, Rapeseed Oil, Cheese Flavour [Dried Cheese (from **Milk**) (7%), **Milk** Lactose, Flavour Enhancer (Disodium 5'-Ribonucleotide), Acid (Lactic Acid), Colours (Paprika Extract, Annatto), Natural Flavourings, Salt, Potassium Chloride]

INGREDIENTS Wholewheat (68%), Dried Fruit (27%) (Raisins, Coconut, Banana {Banana, Coconut Oil, Sugar, Flavouring}, Apple, Hazelnuts), Sugar, Salt, Barley Malt Extract

Manufacturers are still allowed to put additional, voluntary information separately. For example, if the food is produced in a factory that uses any of the top 14 allergens as ingredients in other foods, there is a small risk that tiny amounts of the allergens could get into the food. This is known as cross-contact or cross-contamination. These types of foods are often referred to as 'may contains'.

Unfortunately this type of information is not regulated and so it can be inconsistent between different brands. It is often used as a blanket statement to protect the manufacturer from legal liability. If in doubt, contact the manufacturer directly to ask for more information. You might see a note like one of these:

Not suitable for nut and sesame allergy sufferers due to the methods used in the manufacture of this product.

May contain traces of nuts.

- Contains milk, wheat, gluten, egg
- Recipe: no nuts
- Ingredients: cannot guarantee nut free
- Factory: no nuts

When you are food shopping, allow extra time to read these labels. Check labels of everything you buy, every time, even if your child has eaten it safely before. Manufacturers change their recipes from time to time, and they don't always mark this on the front of the packaging.

When you are starting out, go shopping by yourself. The first time you go shopping it will take you a lot longer as you will need to read every food label thoroughly. This is much more stressful if you also have a small person getting bored and demanding your attention.

Some great apps are available to help when food shopping, such as FoodMaestro, Libereat and SpoonGuru. You can set up a profile with your child's allergies. As you shop, scan product barcodes with your phone and the app will tell you if they are safe or not.

Online shopping is brilliant. You can often get a much bigger range of products than you can find in your local supermarket. You can also take your time reading ingredients, and choose when you want to do it – perhaps when your little one is asleep so you can concentrate. Most online supermarkets will allow you to build up a list of 'favourites' so that you can just shop from products that you know are safe.

You might also see food labelled as 'gluten free'. This means that the food does not have any cereals containing gluten in its ingredients, and is suitable for people on a gluten free diet. By law, the term 'gluten free' can only be used on foods which contain 20 parts per million (ppm) or less of gluten. It does not mean it is suitable for all people with food allergies, only those people who need to avoid gluten. You can see this label on special foods made from gluten substitutes such as breads, biscuits and flour, as well as other foods that are naturally gluten free such as sausages, soups and ready meals.

FREE FROM FOODS

Nowadays, most large supermarkets have a 'Free From' aisle with foods aimed at people with special dietary needs. However, just because something is labelled as 'free from' doesn't mean it will necessarily be safe for your child to eat. You will still need to read the food label carefully. For example, Free From cakes and biscuits may be gluten free, but sometimes still contain milk. Free From bread is also gluten free, but usually contains egg. Dairy free products often contain soya.

It's also important to remember that these special products are made with substitute ingredients. They won't taste exactly the same as the normal version. If you have an older child who is used to eating normal food, they may not like the free from version.

Because they are made with substitute ingredients, they are also heavily processed. This means they may not be as nutritious as normal foods. In addition, they may contain more chemical additives than their regular counterparts. And some foods may have extra sugar or sweetener added to make them taste nicer.

Free from foods are also more expensive than normal foods because they use more expensive ingredients. They can be as much as double or even triple the price, and the portion sizes are often smaller.

For these reasons, it's not a good idea to rely on these 'free from' foods, but to cook from scratch as much as you can, using foods that are naturally safe for your child to eat. However, they are useful for events like parties, so that your child doesn't feel left out, or as a special treat. They can also be useful to help your child get used to the taste and texture of a food, so that if they grow out of their allergy it is easier for you to introduce the real food to their diet e.g. dairy free cheese.

SUBSTITUTE INGREDIENTS

Milk, eggs and wheat are the most difficult ingredients to avoid in cooking. They are staple foods that are used in cooking both sweet and savoury dishes. Luckily nowadays there are many different alternatives available, so there is lots of choice. You can have fun experimenting with different options until you find what your child prefers to eat, and what you prefer to cook with.

Milk alternatives

Each different type of milk alternative has a distinctive taste, so you may need to try a few before you find one that your child likes. They are available plain or in flavoured varieties for drinking. You can get sweetened and unsweetened varieties – choose unsweetened if possible to avoid added sugar or sweeteners. Some brands have added calcium. You can also get fresh or long-life versions.

- Soya milk – this is the closest substitute, if your child can tolerate it. Higher in protein than other milk alternatives.
- Oat milk – some brands are made with gluten free oats, but not all.
- Nut milks – almond milk is the most common, but others such as hazelnut or cashew milk are also available. Made from ground nuts mixed with water.
- Coconut milk drink (not tinned coconut milk) – made by soaking coconut flesh in hot water. The cream is skimmed off the top and the milk is left behind, which is then mixed with water.
- Rice milk – not suitable as a main milk drink for children under 4½ years old as it contains trace amounts of arsenic.
- Hemp milk – made from soaking and grinding hemp seeds mixed with water.
- Tiger nut milk – made from tiger nuts (which are actually a legume, not a nut) and water. Naturally contains calcium.

Cream alternatives

These are similar to the milk alternatives but have a thicker texture, with a similar consistency to single cream. Cream alternatives are usually made from soya, oat or coconut.

Yogurt alternatives

Available as plain or flavoured, yogurt alternatives are most often made from soya or coconut milk. New options are now coming onto the market made from nut or oat milks.

Butter alternatives

- Dairy-free spread e.g. Pure, Vitalite, Flora Dairy Free. Comes in a plastic tub. Use in the same way as butter. No need to soften before using in baking, as it is already soft.
- Dairy-free margarine block e.g. Stork. Comes foil-wrapped. Use as a substitute for butter – not soft like dairy-free spread. Useful for butter icing and pastry.
- Olive oil – good for savoury cooking. Extra-virgin olive oil has a strong flavour and is best saved for salad dressings.
- Rapeseed oil – mild taste, great for baking and very nutritious.
- Sunflower oil – cheap and has many uses.
- Vegetable shortening – useful for making dairy-free pastry.
- Coconut oil – this can be used in baking, sweet recipes, and for cooking things like curry and other savoury recipes. Although it is an oil, it is solid at room temperature. It does have a slight coconutty flavour.

Egg alternatives

In baking, eggs help to bind all the other ingredients together. They also help to make things rise. If you are baking without eggs you can look for vegan recipes which contain no egg and no milk. If you are trying to adapt a normal recipe there are several different egg substitutes you can try.

You can buy commercial egg replacer online, from health food shops and in some supermarkets. Made from a combination of potato flour and tapioca starch, this is a powder that is mixed with water to replace egg in all types of recipes. It can be used for baking and also to make batters, mayonnaise and even meringues. It can be used to replace whole egg, egg white or egg yolk in recipes. Brand names include Orgran Egg Replacer, Free and Easy Egg Replacer and Ener-G Egg Replacer.

For baking there are also some 'natural' egg substitutes. They all have slightly different properties and you may need to use different substitutes in different recipes. The table below shows different ways to substitute one egg.

How to substitute one egg	
Ground flaxseed/linseed	1 tbsp ground flaxseed + 2.5 tbsp water
Chia seeds	1 tbsp chia seeds + 1/3 cup water
Agar agar	1 tbsp agar agar + 1 tbsp water
Ripe bananas	½ mashed banana
Apple puree	¼ cup
Peanut butter	3 tbsp
Soy protein	1 tbsp soy protein powder + 3 tbsp water
Aquafaba (water from tinned chickpeas)	Liquid from one 400ml tin of chickpeas

Wheat flour alternatives

Nowadays, special gluten-free flour mixes are available in nearly every supermarket. These flour mixes can be substituted for normal wheat flour in recipes or used in special gluten free recipes. Other alternatives to wheat flour include:

- Buckwheat flour – despite the name, this has nothing to do with wheat and is actually a seed.
- Gram flour – also known as chickpea flour, this is widely used in Indian cooking.
- Rice flour – this can be used to make shortbread but otherwise not great for baking on its own and needs to be combined with other ingredients.
- Ground rice – this is coarse and usually used for making puddings.
- Masa harina – also known as corn flour, but not the same as cornflour! Can be used to make tortillas.
- Rye flour – doesn't contain wheat, but does contain gluten. This can be used to make bread but it has a very strong taste.
- Coconut flour – high in protein, fibre and healthy fat which makes it very satisfying. It contains many nutrients

as well. It absorbs a lot of liquid and so much less is needed in recipes than other types of flour.

- Ground almonds and almond flour – these are very high in calories, but make gluten free cakes very moist and delicious. Best used in moderation.
- Spelt flour – spelt is closely related to wheat but is not the same. It does contain gluten. Some people who are allergic to wheat can eat spelt but not all. If your child is allergic to wheat, speak to your doctor or dietitian for advice on whether to include spelt in your child's diet.
- Other more unusual flours include amaranth flour, millet flour, quinoa flour, sorghum flour, teff flour and tiger nut flour.

Wheat free grains

These can be used as the starchy part of your meal, to add more variety to your diet. They are can often be found in the free from section of the supermarket or in health food shops. Some of these are pseudo-grains – they are actually a seed. These are actually more nutritious than grains so will have great benefit to your diet. Some of these grains and pseudo-grains may seem exotic but they have actually been eaten by humans for thousands of years.

- Amaranth – pseudo-grain, usually mixed with other types of grain.
- Buckwheat – pseudo-grain. Suitable for salads and risottos. Also available as noodles (soba noodles).
- Maize – polenta or corn. You can also get corn pasta.
- Millet – can be used in soups. Millet flakes can be used to make porridge.
- Oats – oats can be contaminated with gluten due to the way they are processed in factories. However, if your child is allergic to wheat, they may be able to tolerate gluten-free oats, which are processed in a gluten- and wheat-free environment.
- Quinoa – a pseudo grain which looks very similar to cous cous. You can also get quinoa pasta and porridge flakes.
- Rice – there are many different varieties of rice including

basmati, long grain, risotto, paella and short-grain rice (great for making rice pudding). You can also get rice pasta and rice porridge flakes.

Other essentials

These ingredients are not direct substitutes for anything but they are useful in allergy-friendly baking.

- Xanthan gum – brilliant in gluten free baking, helps to bind ingredients together and make the finished result less crumbly. As a general rule, add ½ teaspoon per 100g gluten free plain flour. Gluten free self-raising flour usually has xanthan gum added already.
- Baking powder and bicarbonate of soda – help baked products to rise. If you are baking without eggs, you may need to add extra bicarb or baking powder.
- Arrowroot and cornflour/cornstarch – these can be used to thicken gravies, sauces, soups and stews.

Getting to grips with a food allergy can feel overwhelming at first. Give yourself extra time for food shopping in the first few weeks. Experiment with new foods and find out what your child likes and dislikes. Soon you will find new regular items and favourites and you won't need to give it as much thought. There are new products coming onto the market all the time and the choice is better than ever for people with food allergies.

KEY POINTS

- Always check ingredients carefully when buying food.
- Common allergens must be highlighted in ingredients labels on pre-packed food.
- Food prepared on-site doesn't have to be labelled – you will have to ask for information.
- Cook from scratch whenever possible rather than relying on free-from foods.
- There is a wide range of milk, egg and wheat alternatives – experiment to find which ones you like best.

REFERENCES AND LINKS

- BBC Good Food, 'Glossary' (2018), https://www.bbcgoodfood.com/glossary/a, accessed 10th December 2018.
- Coeliac UK, 'Gluten free product certification' (2018), https://www.coeliac.org.uk/food-industry-professionals/the-crossed-grain-symbol/, accessed 10th December 2018.
- Food Standards Agency, 'Allergen Labelling' (December 2017), https://www.food.gov.uk/business-guidance/allergen-labelling, accessed 10th December 2018.
- Kendrick, Pippa, *The Intolerant Gourmet* (London, 2012).

CHAPTER 5

COOKING AT HOME

Many parents find that the ideal way to manage their child's allergies is to cook from scratch as much as possible. This means you know exactly what ingredients are in their food, you can ensure there is no cross-contact from other ingredients in the kitchen, and it's much cheaper and healthier than relying heavily on packaged foods or ready meals.

AVOIDING CROSS CONTACT

Cross contact (or cross contamination) can occur when different food ingredients are used in the same kitchen. For example, if a chopping board is used to chop different ingredients, the same knife is used to spread butter and jam on different slices of bread, or the same spoon is used to stir different pots of food. As a result, small amounts of the food get mixed together. Even tiny amounts of food that you cannot see could cause an allergic reaction. This is a normal occurrence in most home kitchens, but if your child has allergies you must take steps to avoid it.

How careful you have to be depends on how sensitive your child is. If your child is extremely sensitive and has severe reactions, you may decide to ban the food completely from your home. This obviously will have an effect on all family members. If your child is safe with their food allergen(s) being cooked and eating by other people in the home, you will need to ensure that their food doesn't get contaminated. Here are some suggestions to help you avoid cross contact:

- Store your child's safe foods on a special shelf or in a special cupboard or container. For example, you might keep a separate biscuit tin or bread bin for your child.
- Alternatively, you might keep unsafe foods all together in one place so your child doesn't eat them accidentally.
- Label unsafe foods with red stickers and safe foods with green stickers.
- Do not store 'safe' and 'unsafe' foods next to each other.
- Store foods carefully in the fridge. Keep all foods wrapped or covered.
- Before and after preparing food, clean work surfaces with hot soapy water.
- Before you start cooking, wash your hands with soap and water to remove any traces of food allergens. Note that alcohol-based hand sanitiser does NOT remove food proteins from your hands.
- Wash any utensils, bowls, pots, pans etc in hot soapy water to remove any traces of the food allergen. Just wiping with a cloth does NOT remove food proteins effectively.
- Use separate utensils, pans, chopping boards etc for your child's food. If your child is very sensitive you could buy separate kitchen items that are only ever used for their allergen-free food.
- Avoid contaminating pots of food like jam, yeast extract, butter or margarine. Either use separate utensils whenever taking any food out of these types of containers, or buy separate pots of food for your child and label them.
- When cooking separate foods in the oven, either cook your child's food first on its own, or cook it on the top shelf to prevent drips or crumbs falling into their food.
- If cooking separate meals at the same time, or preparing packed lunches for more than one person, make the allergen free food first.

- Put dirty dishes, cutlery etc. straight into the sink or dishwasher and do not use them again until they have been washed thoroughly.
- Keep safe foods covered and away from unsafe foods to avoid splashes or crumbs.
- If you make a mistake when cooking, throw the food away (or give it to someone else to eat) and start again.
- If your child is very sensitive, teach all family members to wash their hands with soap and water after eating unsafe foods. When guests arrive ask them to wash their hands with soap and water.

By following these steps, you can reduce the risk of cross contact in your home. You may not need to follow all of these steps, again it depends on how sensitive your child is. After a while it will seem like second nature to follow these extra food hygiene steps.

MEAL PLANNING

Weekly meal planning can help in a lot of ways. It requires a little bit of time and organisation but it is very worthwhile. It can help keep your food costs down and reduce food waste as you only buy what you need. You will know in advance what you are going to cook each day and avoid the 5 o'clock what's-for-dinner panic. Doing one big weekly shop, instead of shopping several times a week, is a big timesaver. It can also help you to make sure your child is getting a balanced diet and a good variety of different foods as you can see what they are eating over a week as a whole.

To make a meal plan, you just need to write down what you are going to eat for breakfast, lunch and dinner for a week in advance. Don't forget to include snacks and desserts. Start by asking everyone in the family for their favourite meals, and try to include them in your meal plan. See the next page for an example. A free template is available at www.allergykitchen.com/downloads.

Try to include a good variety of foods in your child's diet, for optimum nutrition. This is even more important if they are on a restricted diet due to food allergies. See if you can include a rainbow of different coloured vegetables and fruits. Think about

MEAL PLAN EXAMPLE (DAIRY AND SOYA FREE)

Day	Breakfast	Snack	Lunch	Snack	Dinner
Mon	Scrambled eggs (no milk or butter) on toast Banana	Apple Rice Cakes	Peanut butter sandwich made with dairy– and soya– free margarine Cucumber slices Coconut milk yogurt	Breadsticks and houmous	Spaghetti Bolognese Rice pudding made with coconut milk
Tue	Crumpets with fruit spread Strawberries	Homemade dairy-free carrot muffins	Dairy– and soya– free pesto pasta with chicken breast Broccoli Fruit puree	Pineapple	Fish fingers with new potatoes, carrots and peas Baked apples with raisins and cinnamon, dairy free custard
Wed	Cornflakes with dairy free milk Banana	Raisins Breadsticks	Jacket potato with tuna and sweetcorn Dairy– and soya– free biscuit	Plain rice cakes with mashed avocado	Homemade pizza with dairy free cheese Baked bananas & chocolate

whether you have included different types of meat such as beef, lamb, pork, chicken, turkey and fish. If you are vegetarian or vegan, try to include a range of different protein sources.

Your meal plan needs to include:

- A variety of vegetables and fruits – aim for at least 5 portions a day. A glass of fruit juice or a smoothie can count as one portion per day, but no more.
- Meals based around starchy foods such as potatoes, rice, pasta or bread. Eat potatoes with skins on and choose wholemeal or brown rice, pasta and bread.
- Dairy, or dairy alternatives fortified with calcium such as soya milk, nut milk, or coconut milk products, or other foods that are naturally high in calcium.
- Protein such as beans, pulses, fish, eggs and meat – aim for two portions of fish per week, including one portion of oily fish.
- Healthy fats in small quantities.

Avoid eating too much of foods with high levels of added sugar, sweeteners and salt, such as biscuits, crisps, chocolate, fizzy drinks, cakes and ice cream. These should only be eaten occasionally and in small amounts. This healthy eating advice is based on current UK Government recommendations.

CALCIUM IN A DAIRY FREE DIET

Cow's milk is most people's main source of calcium, which is needed for healthy bones and teeth. It's also important for muscles, heart health and nerve function. You can get it from products which don't naturally contain calcium, but have it added (calcium-fortified or calcium-enriched products). However, your body can absorb and use calcium from natural sources much more effectively.

Spinach, dried fruits, beans, seeds and nuts are sometimes listed as good sources of calcium. However they also contain oxalate and/or phytates which make the calcium indigestible. This means that although the food contains plenty of calcium, your body will only be able to absorb a small proportion of it.

Naturally calcium rich foods

- Tinned sardines, salmon or pilchards with bones
- Whitebait
- Scampi
- Oranges
- Dark green leafy vegetables
- Broccoli

Calcium fortified products

- Hypoallergenic infant formula or follow-on formula, available on prescription only
- Milk alternatives with added calcium e.g. soya, oat, rice, nut or coconut milk
- White, brown or wholemeal bread have calcium added
- Calcium fortified yogurt, desserts and custard made from milk alternatives e.g. soya, coconut
- Calcium fortified infant cereal
- Calcium fortified breakfast cereal (look for calcium carbonate in the ingredients)
- Calcium fortified instant hot oat cereal e.g. Ready Brek and supermarket own brands
- Soya bean curd/tofu if set with calcium chloride (E509) or calcium sulphate (E516) but not nigari

Notes

- Rice milk should not be given as a main milk drink to children under 4½ years old, as it contains small amounts of arsenic!
- If you are really struggling to get your child to eat enough foods containing calcium, children's calcium supplements are available.
- If you are breastfeeding and on a dairy-free diet, take care

of your own calcium intake as well.

- Vitamin D helps with absorption of calcium, so make sure to remember Vitamin D supplements.

You can also boost how well the body absorbs calcium, to make the most of what your child is getting in their diet.

- Little and often – your body will absorb more calcium if you eat smaller amounts more frequently through the day, rather than having lots all in one go.
- With a meal – your body can absorb calcium more easily if it is part of a meal. If you eat calcium rich foods on their own they may pass through the body too quickly.
- Avoid fizzy drinks – the acid in these drinks actually reduces your body's ability to absorb calcium.
- Combine with Vitamin C-rich foods, such as oranges and orange juice, red and green peppers, strawberries, blackcurrants, broccoli, brussels sprouts and potatoes. Vitamin C helps the body to absorb calcium.
- Get enough Vitamin D – the body also needs vitamin D to absorb calcium so these supplements are even more important for people on a milk free diet.
- Avoid salt and high-protein diets – these can reduce calcium absorption.

SUPPLEMENTS

In addition to eating a balanced, varied diet, the UK Government also recommends that all children aged from 6 months to 5 years old should have vitamin supplements containing Vitamins A, C and D every day. This is because sometimes children don't get enough Vitamin A and C from their diet. In the UK, it is difficult to get enough Vitamin D from food alone, especially in winter (the body usually makes its own Vitamin D from sunshine on the skin).

Breastfed babies are also recommended to have Vitamin D drops from birth to 6 months old. Babies who drink at least 500ml (about a pint) of baby formula a day do not need to have vitamin supplements because formula already contains added vitamins.

Supermarkets and chemists stock many different brands of children's vitamin supplements. They come as drops and chewable tablets or gummies. There are lots of different flavours too, so you should be able to find something that suits your child. Remember to check the ingredients for your child's food allergen(s).

BATCH COOKING

Batch cooking simply means cooking a large batch of food – more than you would normally eat in one sitting – and storing it for another day. This can be as simple as cooking a large batch of bolognese sauce and keeping half for lunch the next day. Most leftovers will keep in the fridge for a few days. You can also freeze your batch of food to keep it for longer. It's like having a stash of your own homemade ready meals on hand. This is a great timesaver because you can cook once and eat twice (or even more).

Batch cooking is particularly handy if you are working. You can still provide home cooked meals by batch cooking on days you are not working, storing them in the fridge or freezer, and then reheating and eating the food on the days you are working. This will save you time, money and stress! It's a great investment of your time, and helps to make weeknights more manageable. Even if you are not working it's still handy for busy days when you are not at home (for example, if you're ferrying children around to after-school clubs and activities) and even those days when you just don't feel like cooking.

This approach can work well for baked goods too. For example, you could make a batch of muffins, freeze them, and then defrost one each day for your child's snack or packed lunchbox. Some people even like to spend one weekend each month preparing, cooking and freezing meals, which they can then eat for the rest of the month. This is know as 'once a month cooking'.

Overleaf are some examples of foods that can be cooked in large batches and frozen. There are many batch cooking recipes available online to help you get started, as well as tips for how to plan and prepare for batch cooking and instructions on freezing food safely and conveniently.

Foods ideal for batch cooking:

- Bolognese sauce
- Curries
- Stews, casseroles and hotpots
- Soups
- Chilis
- Tomato sauce
- Shepherd's pie/cottage pie filling
- Lasagne and other baked pasta dishes
- Quiches
- Pulled pork/lamb/beef
- Ratatouille
- Stuffed peppers
- Veggie burgers
- Fishcakes
- Muffins
- Cakes
- Biscuits
- Scones
- Banana bread
- Granola bars
- Brownies

As a parent of a child with food allergies there's no getting away from it: you will have to put more time and effort into planning and preparing meals. You can't always pop to the corner shop if you run out of something, and it can be difficult to find allergy safe takeaways for days when you are busy or low on energy. However, simple strategies like meal planning and batch cooking can help save you time and effort.

You will also need to consider how you will ensure your child still gets a balanced diet despite their restrictions. This gets easier with time as you build up a repertoire of family meals, and you get into the habit of planning ahead. If you are struggling do not hesitate to seek support from a dietitian – your GP can refer you.

KEY POINTS

- Having a child with food allergies means you will need to cook from scratch most of the time.
- Take care to avoid cross contact in your home kitchen.
- Planning meals can help reduce stress and makes it easier to ensure your family has a balanced diet.
- If your child is allergic to milk, make sure you include plenty of other sources of calcium in their diet.
- Batch cooking can save time in the kitchen.

REFERENCES AND LINKS

- British Dietetic Association, 'Food Fact Sheet: Calcium' (July 2017), https://www.bda.uk.com/foodfacts/Calcium.pdf, accessed 10th June 2018.
- British Nutrition Foundation, 'A healthy, balanced diet' (October 2016), https://www.nutrition.org.uk/healthyliving/healthydiet/healthybalanceddiet.html, accessed 10th June 2018.
- Food Allergy Research & Education, 'Avoiding Cross-Contact' (2018), https://www.foodallergy.org/life-with-food-allergies/living-well-everyday/avoiding-cross-contact, accessed 10th June 2018.
- Kids with Food Allergies, '12 Tips for Avoiding Cross-Contact of Food Allergens' (July 2014), http://www.kidswithfoodallergies.org/page/prevent-allergic-reactions-in-your-home.aspx, accessed 10th June 2018.
- NIH Osteoporosis and Related Bone Diseases National Resource Center, 'Calcium and Vitamin D: Important at Every Age' (May 2015), https://www.bones.nih.gov/health-info/bone/bone-health/nutrition/calcium-and-vitamin-d-important-every-age, accessed 10th June 2018.
- NHS, 'Eating a balanced diet' (March 2016), https://www.nhs.uk/Livewell/Goodfood/Pages/Healthyeating.aspx, accessed 10th June 2018.

- NHS, 'Vitamins for Children' (February 2018),
  https://www.nhs.uk/conditions/pregnancy-and-
  baby/vitamins-for-children/, accessed 10th June 2018.

CHAPTER 6

EATING OUT

Managing your child's food allergies at home is relatively easy as you are in control of the situation. You can make sure the kitchen is clean, and you know exactly what has gone into your child's food. Eating out can be a bit trickier as you have to put your trust in someone else to understand your child's food allergies and provide safe food. Luckily, awareness is growing and with a little bit of planning and organisation it is possible to enjoy eating out even with food allergies.

WHAT IS THE LAW?

In the past, people with food allergies had a very difficult time trying to eat out. They may have been unable to find out for sure whether a food was safe for them to eat or not. They may have been made to feel like an inconvenience, or that they were being fussy. People have even been asked to leave a restaurant because staff were afraid to serve them in case of a reaction. As a result, many people with food allergies didn't eat out at all, or would stick to the same venue and the same food every time they went out.

Thankfully, legislation now provides for people with food allergies so that they can eat out safely. The EU Food Information for Consumers Regulation No. 1169/2011 came into force on 13th

December 2014. This legislation states that food businesses selling unpackaged food, such as restaurants, cafés, cafeterias, deli counters, butchers, bakeries and sandwich bars must provide allergy information. Food businesses must provide information on the same 14 allergens as for packed food sold in shops (see Chapter 4). For cereals containing gluten and nuts, the business must also say which specific cereal or nut is included in the dish.

This allergy information does not have to be given upfront, and you may have to ask to get it. It can be given verbally or in writing and examples of this are covered later in this chapter. However, all businesses must give you this information if you ask for it.

Businesses that don't comply with this regulation will be given an improvement notice by the local authority. If they still don't improve, they will then be given a fine. The size of the fine depends on how big the business is and the impact of the offence – there is no maximum fine. Both businesses and individuals working for the business can be fined. Mislabelling foods containing allergens is a criminal offence, because of the high risk to consumer health and safety. If you have a bad experience, you can find out how to report a problem at the end of this chapter.

Buffet restaurants are more tricky. In a buffet, the information has to be provided for each individual food item separately. However, there is a very high risk of cross-contact in a buffet due to other customers using the same utensils to serve different food, so this is not helpful for very sensitive allergies. You may be able to ask for a fresh plate of food to be made for you in the kitchen, but this is down to the restaurant's discretion.

Free samples are subject to the same legislation, e.g. free samples or tasters, or a free chocolate or biscuit given with a cup of coffee.

Takeaway businesses must also provide allergen information. For example, they may have an online menu with allergen information. Information may be provided verbally over the phone, ideally with a member of staff referring to written information. Containers of food may be labelled with allergen stickers. Or they may deliver a written menu with allergen information along with the food.

ALLERGEN INFORMATION

Current legislation does not say exactly how allergen information must be provided, so there can be a lot of variation between different eating establishments. Here are some examples of what to look out for:

Signposting

You might see a sign on the wall like the one below, which invites you to speak to a member of staff about food allergies. It could be a printed sign, handwritten, or on a chalkboard. The member of staff should be able to provide the information to you verbally, preferably referring to written information, or by checking with the chef. If the business only provides information to customers verbally, they must have a sign inviting people to speak to a member of staff. Here is an example:

FOOD ALLERGIES and INTOLERANCES

Please speak to our staff about the ingredients

in your meal, when placing your order.

Allergen menu spreadsheet

Many restaurants also provide a more detailed allergen menu in the form of a spreadsheet. These give you more information but are often written in very small writing and can be harder to read. Here is a partial example:

Menu Item	Celery	Cereals containing Gluten	Eggs	Fish	Milk
Vegetable Crudites with Garlic Bread	No	Yes, Wheat	Yes	No	Yes
Pasta with Tomato Sauce	Yes	Yes, Wheat	No	No	No
Pasta Carbonara	Yes	Yes, Wheat	Yes	No	Yes
Cheese and Tomato Pizza	No	Yes, Wheat	No	No	Yes

Menu with symbols

Allergen information is sometimes included within the normal menu which is given to all customers. This may include letters or symbols to show which allergens are present in the food, for example:

~ MAINS ~

Chicken goujons with chips, peas and sweetcorn G E D C M S

Beef burger with chips G E D SO N M S

Sausages and mash with peas and sweetcorn G D C SD

Pasta with tomato sauce G D

~ ALLERGENS KEY ~

G: Cereals containing Gluten
E: Egg
D: Dairy
C: Celery
SO: Soya
N :Nuts
M: Mustard
S: Sesame
SD: Sulphur Dioxide (sulphites)

Full ingredients listing

Some restaurants go above and beyond what is required by the law and provide a full ingredients listing for each item on the menu, in addition to detailed allergen information. This would usually be provided in a large folder, which takes time to look through but is great if you need to adapt a dish, or have an allergy that is not covered by the legislation. Here is an example extract:

Kid's Chicken Burger			
Ingredients: Chicken breast fillet, marinade (spirit vinegar, rapeseed oil, spice blend (salt, cayenne, hot red paprika, chilli), garlic puree, lemons, green chillies, water), bread roll (see separate page for ingredients), mayonnaise (see separate page), tomato slice, lettuce leaf, basting sauce (see separate page).			
Contains	**Yes**	**No**	**Comments**
Nuts & Derivatives		✓	
Peanuts & Derivatives		✓	
Fish & Derivatives		✓	
Eggs & Derivatives	✓		Bread roll & mayonnaise contain eggs
Crustaceans		✓	
Molluscs		✓	
Milk & derivatives	✓		Bread roll contains milk
Soya & derivatives	✓		Bread roll contains soya

BENEFITS OF THE LEGISLATION

Food businesses are becoming more aware of the needs of people with food allergies. Allergy sufferers feel more confident about asking staff for information, because they know it is required by law. People's knowledge and awareness is improving, although there is a lot of variation between establishments. The biggest improvement has been in provision for gluten free and nut free people, as there is generally a higher level of understanding for these two specific allergies.

WHAT THE LEGISLATION DOES NOT COVER

Food businesses have to tell you what's in your food, but don't have to provide food that is free from any of the allergens. However, many companies are realising that this is good business due to the rise in people with special diets. For example, in some restaurants you may see special gluten free menus, and vegan menus are becoming more common too – these will be free from dairy and egg. However, by law businesses are only required to tell you what you can't eat and are not required to provide you with any alternative.

Companies also don't have to give you a full ingredients list, so if your child has an unusual allergy that is not one of the top 14, you may need to be more persistent to get the information you need.

Businesses have to give the allergy information for the final dish as served, and not for each component of a dish. This can make it tricky to work out what you actually can eat. Some businesses do provide this additional information voluntarily, which can help you to adapt a dish to suit your child's needs. For example, if you needed to avoid wheat, you could ask for a hot dog without a bun, as long as the sausage is wheat-free.

Current legislation does not make any specific provision for training staff about food allergies, so knowledge and understanding does vary a lot between different places. However, all staff in food service must have basic training in food hygiene.

PLANNING TO EAT OUT

Sadly, having food allergies does make it more difficult to be spontaneous. You do need to plan ahead to minimise the risk of accidental exposure. However, there are some simple steps you can follow to make sure a venue is safe for your child to eat at, so you can still enjoy a meal out if you want to. You may want to:

- Use apps such as Biteappy and Libereat to find possible places to eat.
- Check the website – many restaurants (especially chains) provide an allergen menu online. Otherwise, you may be able to look at the normal menu and find some possible safe options.
- Look at review websites such as TripAdvisor or the venue's Facebook page. This can give you a general idea about hygiene and service standards. Look for reviews from previous customers with special dietary requirements.
- Phone ahead and speak to staff. Ask if they are able to cater for your child's food allergies, find out what food choices they are able to provide, and book a specific meal preference if necessary. If they aren't able to provide suitable food, ask if you can bring your own safe food for your child.
- Go into the restaurant ahead of time and speak to staff face to face (as above).

- Check the menu in the window/outside to identify possible safe options.
- When you arrive at the venue, ask if they have an allergen menu.
- When ordering the food, make sure to tell the staff about your child's allergies. If necessary (if your child has severe allergies) explain about cross-contact and the need to cook the food separately.
- To help you when talking to staff about your child's allergies, download and print out allergy cards to give to the person serving you: https://www.food.gov.uk/sites/default/files/allergy-chef-cards.pdf
- Double check the food is safe when it arrives by asking the server if the order is correct, look at the food carefully, and if necessary taste test a small amount.
- Check that the restaurant is safe and hygienic in general and that food is fresh – general good food hygiene is a positive sign of an underlying level of care.
- If any point you are unsure if the venue or food is safe, don't be afraid to make a fuss, or leave!

WHAT TO EXPECT WHEN EATING OUT

Eating out with food allergies is a little bit different. Your child may only have one safe choice for their meal in a particular restaurant. This is likely to be something simple like pasta with tomato sauce, chicken and chips or jacket potato. Some restaurants do offer gluten free pasta, gluten free pizza and even dairy free pizza (with vegan cheese). Dessert might be jelly, an ice lolly, sorbet or fruit salad. Be prepared that your child may be disappointed if someone in your group is eating something they like but aren't allowed. You can always offer to make this food at home for their next meal.

If the restaurant you want to visit doesn't have anything suitable on the menu, they may be able to adapt an existing meal. Alternatively, you may be able to bring food from home, so that your child can still join in with the social side of eating out.

It may take longer to order your meal as you will need to ask questions. Staff may need extra time to check ingredients by talking to the chef, referring to written information or checking food packaging. It may also take a bit longer to cook your food if they have to cook it separately and change utensils and so on.

A good tip is to visit restaurants outside of busy times, when waiting staff will have more time to talk to you and kitchen staff will be less rushed. This reduces the chance of mistakes being made.

WHAT PROBLEMS DO PEOPLE STILL EXPERIENCE?

The new legislation has been a huge help in raising awareness of food allergies and making it safer for people with food allergies to eat out. Staff in eating venues generally have a much more positive attitude to people with food allergies. However, people do still experience some problems when they try to eat out. For example:

- Restaurants refusing to provide any food for a person with a food allergy because they are scared of a reaction.
- Being over cautious and labelling everything as 'may contain' meaning there is nothing safe to eat.
- Allergen menus being out of date or having incorrect information.
- Poor understanding of allergies, such as thinking that eggs are dairy, confusing lactose intolerance and milk allergy, or thinking that gluten free foods are suitable for anyone with any allergy.
- Allergen information being difficult to read e.g. in a large spreadsheet of data printed with tiny writing.
- Casual staff may have a lack of knowledge and understanding of allergies.
- Bringing incorrect food, and then simply scraping the allergen off the top and giving the food back, rather than making up a new plate of food.
- Removing items from a dish to make it safe, but not providing any replacement, meaning you end up with a smaller portion of food but still pay full price.

- In some chain restaurants, all the food is pre-prepared and the staff just reheat it, so menu items cannot be changed.
- Staff not speaking English well enough to communicate properly.
- No understanding of cross contact in the restaurant kitchen or how to prevent it.

WHAT TO DO IF SOMETHING GOES WRONG

There are a number of steps you can take if you are not happy with the service provided with regard to food allergies. It's important to speak up because it is a matter of health and safety, for your own child and for anyone else with food allergies who comes to that venue in future.

- Speak to staff at the premises – talk to the server or ask to speak to the chef or manager about the importance of getting it right.
- Complain on their social media – this is useful if they are providing allergen information, but don't provide any suitable alternative foods and don't allow you to bring your own food – simply excluding people with food allergies.
- Leave a bad review on sites such as TripAdvisor or apps like Biteappy and Libereat. This helps future visitors and might also spur the restaurant on to make changes!
- Report them to the local authority's Environmental Health department – they are responsible for inspecting venues and enforcing the law. You can do this at https://www.food.gov.uk/enforcement/report-problem
- Report them to Trading Standards via the Citizen's Advice consumer helpline on 03454 040506 or online.

Understandably, people with food allergies do tend to eat out less often than those without food allergies. However, by taking precautions you should still be able to enjoy eating out from time to time. By law, restaurants and cafes are required to give you information about allergens in the food. Plan ahead as much as possible and always tell staff about your child's food allergies when ordering food.

KEY POINTS

- Plan ahead when eating out.
- Food businesses must provide you with information about what allergens are in their food if you ask for it, by law.
- Food service staff may not have a good understanding of food allergies. Ask to speak to a manager if necessary.
- If in doubt, leave! Don't risk it.

REFERENCES AND LINKS

- Food Standards Agency, 'Allergen Labelling' (December 2017),
  https://www.food.gov.uk/enforcement/regulation/fir, accessed 14th November 2018.
- Food Standards Agency, 'Food allergen labelling and information requirements under the EU Food Information for Consumers Regulation No. 1169/2011: Technical Guidance' (April 2015),
  https://www.food.gov.uk/sites/default/files/food-allergen-labelling-technical-guidance.pdf, accessed 14th November 2018.
- Food Standards Agency, 'Preferences for consumers with food allergies or intolerances when eating out' (July 2017),
  https://www.food.gov.uk/research/food-allergy-and-intolerance-research/preferences-for-consumers-with-food-allergies-or-intolerances-when-eating-out, accessed 14th November 2018.
- Hines, Tony, 'Will the UK Sentencing Guidelines Improve Allergen Labelling?', *Leatherhead Food Research* (2016),
  https://www.leatherheadfood.com/files/2016/08/White-Paper-Will-the-UK-Sentencing-Guidelines-Improve-Allergen-Labelling.pdf, accessed 14th November 2018.

CHAPTER 7

TRAVELLING WITH FOOD ALLERGIES

Studies have shown that families with a child with food allergies often take fewer holidays. They may only travel within their own country, or avoid travelling by plane or boat. Although there is a chance of having an allergic reaction when travelling with food allergies, the good news is there are steps you can take to greatly reduce the risk so that travel is still possible and safe. There is no need to let your child's food allergies hold you back if you enjoy travelling. A handy safe travel checklist is provided at the end of this chapter.

CHOOSING A DESTINATION

Travel within the UK has a lot of advantages – you'll have access to familiar supermarkets, brands and restaurants which makes it much easier to find safe foods. There is no language barrier. It can also mean a shorter travel time and is often cheaper than travelling abroad.

You might also consider travelling within the EU, as they have the same labelling laws as we do in the UK. This means that all the top allergens will be highlighted in bold on food packaging, and restaurants have to provide information on what allergens are in their food (see Chapters 4 and 6). Many other countries also have similar labelling laws, but the specific allergens that must be listed vary from country to country.

Think about the local culture when you are choosing a destination. For example, Thai food uses a lot of peanuts, soya is a key ingredient in Chinese food and Indian food often contains nuts and milk. It may be very difficult to avoid these allergens in these countries, unless you are prepared to cook all your own food.

A good place to start is the website Allergy Travels which reviews countries and airlines for allergy-friendliness, and also has a forum where you can connect with other travellers with allergies. The International Food Allergy & Anaphylaxis Alliance has developed specific travel tips for different countries (search online for 'IFAAA travel tips'). Facebook groups for those with food allergies can also be a good source of recommendations.

CHOOSING ACCOMMODATION

Self-catering accommodation offers you the most control and flexibility as you can bring food with you to cook while you are away, and even your own kitchen utensils and equipment if you prefer. You can clean the kitchen when you arrive if necessary. You can also research other dining options at your destination to give you the option of eating out.

All-inclusive resorts may be another option for those with food allergies. Rather than needing to find a new restaurant every meal and explain from scratch each time, you will only have one set of staff to communicate with. Be sure you call ahead and speak to the manager to let them know about your child's allergies and specific needs.

Choose a resort or hotel where at least one member of staff speaks English. Don't assume that because one eating venue in a resort is safe, they all are. Ask about ingredients every time. Also remember that different staff will be on duty at different times. If you've stayed at a resort in the past and had a good experience, remember that things can change over time so make sure to recheck before visiting again.

EATING SAFELY ABROAD

If you are travelling to a non-English speaking country, bring translation cards explaining your child's food allergies. You can buy durable plastic ones from the charity Allergy UK or you can print your own for free on the website Allergy Action. Or download an allergy translation app like AllergyMe Translate or AssureTech.

When shopping in non-English supermarkets, stick to unprocessed food such as meat, fish, vegetables, fruit, rice and potatoes. In restaurants, choose simple foods without sauces and dressing. Before you leave, make sure you know what your allergen is in the native language. If it is a country with a different alphabet, take a picture of it on your phone so you can match it to food packaging.

FLYING

Severe allergic reactions (anaphylaxis) during flights are very rare, but when they do happen the consequences can be worse because you cannot get to hospital facilities quickly. There are several steps you can take to reduce the risk of a reaction whilst flying. Some of these steps may also apply when travelling by boat or train.

There is no legislation covering flying and food allergies in the UK. As a result, there is a lot of variation between airlines. You can check airlines' allergy policies online. Some airlines may be able to provide a special meal (although these are factory produced and cannot be guaranteed to be allergen free). Otherwise you will need to bring your own food for the flight – this is the safest option.

For nut and peanut allergies, you may be able to find an airline that doesn't serve snacks containing nuts/peanuts, but remember that other passengers may still bring them aboard. Some airlines will allow you to book a 'buffer zone' where people near you will be asked not to eat nuts/peanuts. Other airlines will announce that there is a person with a nut/peanut allergy on board and ask other passengers not to eat them. Otherwise, if you politely explain to the passengers sitting near you that your child has a severe allergy then most people will be very understanding.

Communication is the most important factor to ensure safety. Inform the airline of your child's allergy at the time of booking. Contact them again about a week before flying to confirm. Try to get any special accommodations in writing, and bring them with you to the airport. Remind the staff of your requests at check-in, at the gate, and when boarding the plane. Arrive early at the airport to allow extra time to do this. Book a direct flight if possible, so that you only have one team of flight attendants to deal with. Remember to make the same arrangements for connecting and return flights.

Many airlines will allow people with severe allergies to pre-board the plane to wipe down the seats, tray and armrests. You may need a letter from your doctor, depending on the airline's policy. You can also buy disposable seat covers as an extra precaution, or bring a fitted sheet to cover the seat. Don't allow your child to put their hands in the seatback pockets as they could contain food crumbs. Book an early morning flight if you can, as staff will have more time to clean the plane at the end of the day, rather than in-between flights when they may be in a rush. This reduces the chances of coming into contact with crumbs or food residue.

When you need to clean your hands, use wipes or, better still, wash with soap and water in the toilets. Remember that hand gel sanitiser does not get rid of food allergens. You should also avoid using airline pillows and blankets, which could be contaminated with food residue.

Try to seat your child away from other passengers, e.g. in between you and your partner, or in a window seat. When reserving your flight, request the back or front row of a section, which will keep you away from other passengers.

Bring a letter or emergency care plan signed by your child's doctor, or a copy of your child's prescription, to show airport security personnel for your child's medications. Take photos of any documentation and your child's medication on your phone just in case it gets lost, and keep an additional copy in your checked luggage. During the flight, if your child has an epinephrine auto-injector, keep it close to you and not in the overhead locker. Some airlines carry epinephrine, and a few carry auto-injectors, but this cannot be relied upon.

The safest option for eating on the flight is to bring your own food. Bring non-perishable food as most airlines cannot store or reheat passengers' own food. If you have a stopover in another country as part of your journey, check local regulations, as some countries do not allow certain types of food in transit.

A 2013 study found that, for nut and peanut allergy sufferers, these seven steps can massively reduce the chances of having an allergic reaction on board a plane:

1. Requesting special accommodations before the flight.
2. Requesting a peanut/tree nut-free meal.
3. Wiping down the tray table.
4. Avoiding airline pillows and blankets.
5. Requesting a 'buffer zone'.
6. Requesting other passengers not consume peanut/tree nut-containing products.
7. Not eating airline food.

Greenhawt, M., MacGillivray, F., Batty, G., Said, M. and Weiss, C. "International Study of Risk-Mitigating Factors and In-Flight Allergic Reactions to Peanut and Tree Nut" *The Journal of Allergy And Clinical Immunology: In Practice* 1.2 (2013)

SAFETY PRECAUTIONS

Careful planning and research will minimise chances of your child coming into contact with their allergen(s) while travelling. However, you do need to be prepared for a reaction just in case.

Bring all of your child's allergy medication such as antihistamines, inhalers and epinephrine auto-injectors. Check the expiry date of any medication well before you leave and order more if necessary. Keep the medication with you at all times. Make sure every adult in your group knows the signs of an allergic reaction and how to give the medication.

If your child needs an auto-injector, always carry two with you, and consider having more in your luggage. Store your auto-injectors in an insulated bag to maintain a temperature between 20-25C. Do not expose them to heat or direct sunlight, or put them in a refrigerator.

You might also want your child to wear a special bracelet or clothing that shows they have allergies, especially if your child will be away from you in a kids' club or other childcare. These can be bought cheaply on eBay and from other websites.

Find out how to contact emergency services in the country you are visiting. Find out where the nearest hospital accident and emergency department is just in case of a reaction. Take your mobile phone, and make sure you can use it abroad before you leave.

Make sure you have travel insurance that covers medical costs, as emergency hospital care can be expensive. Check that the insurance covers allergic reactions. Some companies offer specialist insurance for people with severe allergies.

Travelling with food allergies is perfectly possible as long as you take precautions. If you enjoy seeing the world, it is well worth the extra effort. Overleaf is a safe travel checklist for you to refer to if you are planning a trip.

KEY POINTS

- When travelling, plan ahead thoroughly – research accommodation, travel arrangements, local supermarkets, restaurants and medical services.
- Allergen translation cards or apps are useful when travelling abroad.
- Take steps to reduce the chances of an allergic reaction when flying.
- Remember to bring all your child's medication and documentation.
- Bring plenty of food for the journey – more than you think you will need.

SAFE TRAVEL CHECKLIST

This checklist is provided for guidance only.

A printable version is available from
www.myallergykitchen.com/downloads

✓	
	Inform hotel/resort of allergies.
	Inform airline of allergies. • Request allergen-free meal if applicable • Request other special accommodations if needed
	Pack enough safe snacks, food and drinks for the trip. • Pack snacks for the journey, plus extra in case of delays. • Pack enough for the whole trip if you are unsure whether safe foods will be available. • Store perishable foods in a suitable coolbox.
	Pack allergen translation cards to use in shops and restaurants, and/or download an app or save useful words/phrases to your phone.
	Other items to pack: • Hand wipes. • Mobile phone & charger. • Travel pillow and blanket for flight.
	Medical items to pack: • Auto-injectable epinephrine (at least 2 doses, preferably 4) in travel cases. • Antihistamines. • Inhalers and any other asthma medications. • Medical ID bracelet/wristband. • Emergency action plan or letter, signed by doctor.
	Take photos of all medical documentation on your phone.
	Check method for calling emergency services at your destination.
	Check location of nearest emergency hospital department.
	Check location of nearest supermarkets.
	Contact local restaurants to see if they can cater for your child's allergies.

REFERENCES AND LINKS

- Allergic Living, 'Comparing Airlines' (March 2016), https://allergicliving.com/wp-content/uploads/2010/08/Comparing-Airlines-Chart-2016_MAR15_V3.pdf, accessed 23rd October 2018.

- Anaphylaxis Campaign, 'Travelling Advice and Tips' (n.d.), https://www.anaphylaxis.org.uk/living-with-anaphylaxis/travelling/holiday-top-tips/ , accessed 23rd October 2018.

- Dolan, Cathy, 'Food Allergies and Flying', *Allergy Lifestyle* (May 2018), https://www.allergylifestyle.com/food-allergies-and-flying/ , accessed 23rd October 2018.

- Food Allergy Research & Education, 'All-Inclusive Resorts' (n.d.), https://www.foodallergy.org/life-with-food-allergies/managing-lifes-milestones/traveling/all-inclusive-resorts, accessed 23rd October 2018.

- Food Allergy Research & Education, 'Before You Head to the Airport' (n.d.), https://www.foodallergy.org/life-with-food-allergies/managing-lifes-milestones/traveling/before-you-head-to-the-airport, accessed 23rd October 2018.

- International Air Transport Association, 'Allergen-Sensitive Passengers (December 2016), https://www.iata.org/whatwedo/safety/health/Documents/allergen-sensitive-passenger.pdf , accessed 23rd October 2018.

- International Food Allergy & Anaphylaxis Alliance, 'Travel Plan of the IFAAA' (n.d.), https://www.foodallergy.org/sites/default/files/migrated-files/file/IFAAA-Travel-Plan.pdf , accessed 23rd October 2018.

- Kids with Food Allergies, 'People with Peanut/Tree Nut Allergies Can Minimize Risk of Reactions on Airplane Flights' (March 2013), https://community.kidswithfoodallergies.org/blog/peanut-nut-allergy-risk-flying-airplanes-allergic-reaction, accessed 23rd October 2018.

- Sánchez-Borges M, Cardona V, Worm M, Lockey RF, Sheikh A, Greenberger PA, Ansotegui IJ, Ebisawa M, El-

Gamal Y, Fineman S, Geller M, Gonzalez-Estrada A, Tanno L, and Thong BY, 'In-flight allergic emergencies', *World Allergy Organization Journal*, 10, 15 (2017) doi: 10.1186/s40413-017-0148-1

CHAPTER 8

CHILDCARE AND SCHOOL

Starting with a childminder or nursery and going to school are big milestones for any child. But it can be especially nerve-wracking if your child has food allergies, as you will be relying on other people to keep your child safe. You can't control everything that happens to your child, but what you can do is set up a food allergy management plan. This will minimise the risk of a reaction and make sure that adults who have responsibility for your child know what to do in the event of a reaction. You must also ensure your child is included in activities as much as possible. The social aspect of school is so important and you don't want your child to be isolated because of their allergies.

Children with food allergies have additional needs, but they are not ill in the usual sense of the word. They are normal children in every respect, except for when they come into contact with a particular food. They need additional care to keep them safe, and to make sure they are fully included in all parts of the day. There are laws in place to protect your child's rights – this is not optional.

Children at different ages and stages have different needs in terms of managing food allergies. Babies and toddlers put things in their mouths and also crawl or play on the floor. Even preschool children put their hands in their mouth a lot. Very young children may not be able to say if they are having a reaction. At primary school age, children want to fit in with their peers. At secondary school age, teenagers become more independent, but they are also more likely to take risks (see Chapter 12). It's important to adapt how you manage your child's allergies as they grow and develop.

CHILDMINDERS

Childminders are individuals who look after other people's children in their own home for payment. Childminders provide a family style, homely environment to look after children. They may work on their own, with another childminder, or employ an assistant. Childminders must be registered with OFSTED and follow the Early Year Foundation Stage (EYFS) Statutory Framework. They can look after up to six children under the age of eight. Up to three of these children can be under five, and only one can be under the age of one year. This includes the childminder's own children if they are under the age of eight.

Childminders must follow the EU Food Information for Consumers Regulation No. 1169/2011 and provide information on food allergens in any food they provide, in the same way that restaurants and cafés do (see Chapter 6). This could be in writing or verbally, but they must have written records that can be checked and provide signposting, such as a poster on the wall inviting you to ask for information about allergens.

The EYFS states that providers must obtain information about children's food allergies and special health requirements before they start attending the setting. They must have a system in place to ensure that children with an allergy or intolerance are not given food containing that allergen. They must keep a record of any information you give them about your child's dietary needs and act on this information.

NURSERY OR PRESCHOOL

Nursery and preschool settings provide more formal, group childcare and early education. They may be privately run, attached to a school or run by a charity. They have different staff ratios to childminders, and each adult will have more children to look after, with multiple members of staff in each setting. Each child will have a named 'key person' who is responsible for looking after that child, and they will be the main person you speak to on a day-to-day basis.

Age	Minimum Staff Ratio
Under 2	1 carer for every 3 children
2-3 years	1 carer for every 4 children
3-5 years	1 carer for every 8 children

As with childminders, nurseries and preschools must follow the EU regulations and provide information about food allergens in any food they serve in the setting. If they offer meals they may have a menu you can look at, or a full set of recipes listing all ingredients. They must also get information from parents about children's food allergies and have a plan in place to prevent a reaction. Staff should take steps to avoid cross contact. All staff should be made aware of individual children's dietary needs. They must also make sure that children with special dietary needs are included in meal and snack times.

SCHOOLS

The Children and Families Act 2014 Section 100 states that all, schools have a duty to support pupils with medical conditions, so that they can have full access to education, including school trips and physical education. They must be supported in terms of their physical and mental health. This legislation includes children with food allergies.

The school does not have to wait for formal diagnosis before providing support to pupils. Waiting lists for referral to a specialist can be long and so the school should make adjustments if food allergies are suspected. Any special arrangements that are needed should be put in place so that they are ready when the child starts school. If the child changes school in the middle of a term or has a new diagnosis, then arrangements should be made within two weeks.

Schools cannot prevent children from joining in with any aspect of school life. They cannot make up rules that make it more difficult for children to join in, such as requiring parents of a child with food allergies to come on trips. Of course, you are allowed to go with your child on a trip if you want, but it should not be a requirement. Ideally, a member of staff should carry out a risk assessment before any special activities and talk to the child, parents and healthcare professionals beforehand as appropriate.

CHOOSING A SETTING

When you are looking around a setting for the first time, talk to the staff about food allergies. Find out what they know about food allergies, including how to prevent cross-contact, and whether they have ever looked after a child with food allergies before. Do they have a food allergy policy? There can be a lot of variation in knowledge and understanding of allergies, depending on people's previous experience. You need to find somewhere that is willing to work with you to keep your child safe and well.

POTENTIAL FOOD ALLERGENS IN CHILDCARE AND SCHOOL SETTINGS

Meal and snack times are the most obvious risk for coming into contact with allergens. There are some other activities that might also be a risk for your child, depending on their individual needs. Make sure your child's carer or teacher is aware if any of these are a potential problem, so that your child can be included safely in all activities.

- Birthday or special occasion celebrations involving food.
- Counting or sorting with beans, pasta, grains, sweets or other small foods.
- Sensory tables that use grains, pasta, sweets or other small foods, or wet foods such as custard, porridge or jelly.
- Arts and crafts projects using food containers such as egg cartons, milk cartons, drinks cartons, yogurt pots and so on.
- Play kitchen or home corner with real food containers.

- Musical instruments – mouth blown instruments may be contaminated.
- Hand washing soap may contain allergens.
- Cloth hand towels may be contaminated with allergens.
- Finger paint, play dough and other craft supplies may contain food allergens.
- Gardening activities such as making bird feeders or planting seeds may be a risk for contact with food allergens.

FOOD ALLERGY MANAGEMENT PLAN

Some school and childcare settings may already have food allergy policies. You will need to make sure they also have a written allergy management plan for your individual child. This might also be called an individual healthcare plan. This is particularly important if your child has severe allergies. Psychologically, people take things that are written down more seriously and see them as more important. Verbal agreements can easily be forgotten.

The allergy management plan will need to include some or all of the following information, as appropriate:

- Exactly what food(s) your child is allergic to.
- Signs and symptoms of a reaction.
- Medicines, when to give them and what dosage.
- Exactly what accommodations your child needs to prevent an allergic reaction, whilst ensuring that they can be fully included in all aspects of the day.
- What your child can do themselves e.g. refusing food offered by another child.
- What support your child needs e.g. supervision at mealtimes.
- Who needs to be aware of your child's allergies.
- Which staff will be available to provide support.
- Staff training required e.g. auto-injector training.
- Additional support around educational, emotional and social needs e.g. tackling allergy bullying.

- What to do in an emergency, including who to contact.
- Practical requirements such as hand washing and seating arrangements.
- Managing school trips and other special activities.

Ensure that your child's allergy management plan is reviewed every year. The plan should also be reviewed if your child does have a reaction at school. Also remember to tell the school if your child grows out of any of their allergies so they can update the plan.

MEETING THE STAFF

Arrange a meeting with your child's teacher or carer to discuss their food allergies and set up a food allergy management plan. You might also want to involve the manager (in a nursery or preschool), headteacher, or SENCO (special educational needs coordinator, in a school setting). Before the meeting, it can be helpful to send everyone who is coming a list of key points that you would like to cover. This gives everyone a chance to prepare, and you'll know that you haven't missed anything.

Remember that members of staff will need time to learn things that have become second nature to you, such as planning food very carefully and reading food labels. They may also be unaware of how isolating food allergies can be.

Approach the school/setting with a positive attitude and aim to create trust between you and the staff with good communication between everyone involved. Do this as early as you can so that the school/setting has time to make any changes, ask questions and get everything ready – including training staff – *before* your child starts. Work together with them to find solutions to any problems. Ongoing communication is key, and you may need to keep reminding teachers or key workers, as allergies are easily forgotten when you don't have to live with them on a daily basis.

MEDICATION

You will need to provide the school with any medication your child needs, both on a regular basis and in an emergency, such as:

- Epinephrine auto-injector x2
- Oral antihistamines and measuring spoon
- Asthma inhaler
- Eczema creams

Make sure you also give the school any documentation that goes with the medication and instructions on how to use it. Emphasise that it if there is any doubt, it is better to give the medication than to wait and see.

Epinephrine auto-injectors should be stored close by, ideally in the classroom, in an unlocked cupboard so that they can be quickly and easily accessed in case of an emergency. If your child is taking part in activities outside of the classroom, e.g. sports activities on the school field, they should still have rapid access to their medication and someone who is trained to use it. This means it should be taken with them, wherever they are going.

REDUCING EXPOSURE TO ALLERGENS

Here are some suggestions of special accommodations you may want to ask for to reduce your child's exposure to allergens. These adjustments are simple and inexpensive, but will make all the difference in keeping your child safe. Remember that your child is an individual so you need to do what is best for them.

- Keep a container of safe sweets to use as rewards/treats, or have non-food items like stickers, pencils or small toys.
- All children to wash hands before *and after* eating or handling food. Baby wipes are also ok for cleaning hands, but antibacterial hand gel does not remove food proteins.
- Avoid use of allergens in class projects, parties, holidays and celebrations, arts, crafts, science experiments, cooking, snacks or rewards.
- Wash tables, chairs and any other eating areas before *and after* each meal and snack.
- Safe seating arrangements, such as having a peanut table for anyone with peanuts in their lunch – remembering it is always better to exclude the food and not the child. Your

child should always be socialising as normally as possible and never sitting by themselves to eat.

- Keep eating areas separate from learning/playing areas.
- Store food carefully and prepare food safely to prevent cross-contact.
- Keep a photo of your child with a reminder of their allergies stuck on the wall in a place where members of staff can see it e.g. in the school office, in the staff room, in the cafeteria and/or in the classroom.
- For birthdays and other celebrations, only allow pre-packaged food with ingredients labels rather than homemade.
- Ask for a written letter to be sent home to all parents explaining that there is a child with food allergies in the class and what they can do to help (you can offer to write this letter).

EMPOWERING YOUR CHILD

It's really important to teach your child about their food allergies so that they can advocate for themselves when you are not there. As they grow up they need to learn as much as they can about their food allergies and keeping themselves safe. They need to know exactly what food(s) they are allergic to, and that ingredients can be hidden inside foods. Teach them never to take food from anyone except you. They should also know what medication they have and what it is for (including auto-injectors, oral antihistamines and inhalers) and where it is stored. They also need to be able to tell an adult if they feel unwell, when they are old enough to do this.

Remember though, that this is an ongoing process, and it will depend on your child's age and level of understanding. Children do make mistakes – for example, young children love to share food and may be persuaded by a friend to eat different food. Don't be cross with them, just remind them of the importance of avoiding their allergen(s) to keep them safe.

It may also help if your child wears a medical bracelet with their allergy information written on it. This is a great visual reminder to other people and can alert different staff to your child's allergies who might not normally be aware, such as specialist subject teachers or supply teachers. You can also buy lunchboxes with allergy alerts printed on them which can be useful for younger children.

SCHOOL DINNERS VS PACKED LUNCHES

Many parents of children with food allergies prefer to send their child with a packed lunch. This is absolutely the safest option. School dinner provision varies a lot between schools. Some schools still have a traditional kitchen with food cooked on site. If this is the case, you can meet with the cook and discuss your child's needs. Other schools have school dinners cooked off-site by a catering firm. They are still required to provide you with allergen information, but it can be more difficult to build the trust that they will provide safe food for your child.

Some schools are already 'nut free', including school dinners. They may also provide a 'non-gluten-containing-ingredients' menu, which is a label used when the caterer cannot guarantee that there is no cross contact in the kitchen. Many schools will make school dinners allergy safe just by removing the allergen in question, and not replacing it with anything else. This is especially the case with milk. For example, they may have pasta bake without the cheese topping, or chicken curry with no yogurt. They may be provided with puddings with no custard, or just a plain biscuit or fruit each day. In this case, you might be able to send your child with their own dairy-free custard or yogurt if you want to.

Even if you decide to give your child packed lunches, it is always worth investigating the options and having plans put in place. That way, if your child did need to have school dinners in an emergency, kitchen staff will already be aware of their needs and they would be able to provide a safe lunch, even if it is just a jacket potato.

BE A PROACTIVE PARENT

As an allergy parent, it's even more important than usual to build a good relationship with your child's school, nursery or childminder and keep channels of communication open. You can volunteer to help at special occasions such as parties and celebrations or join the PTA and help out with fundraising events such as fetes and cakes sales. This way you'll have advance notice of what's going on, and being involved at the planning stage means you can help to make sure things are safe. This is particularly helpful in the beginning so you can identify any potential problems. You are the expert on your child's allergies.

You may want to provide your child's teacher with a list of safe treats, or give them a special box filled with treats for your child to give as rewards or for celebrations. It can also be helpful to give your child's teacher some extra snacks to keep just in case of an emergency, for example if they drop their lunch on the floor!

It's really important to take the time to set up arrangements for your child to keep them safe while they are in someone else's care. If you set up a good food allergy management plan and communicate openly with your child's teacher or carer, your child will be well taken care of. At the same time, you will be helping to raise awareness of allergies which will help not only your child but also anyone else with food allergies who comes to the nursery or school in future. It can be really beneficial to teach all children in a setting about food allergies, as young children love to help look after each other. This will help everyone to have better understanding of diversity and the different needs of all children.

KEY POINTS

- Children with food allergies need extra care at childminders, nurseries, preschools and schools.
- Staff must take steps to ensure your child is both safe and included in activities.
- Teach your child how to keep themselves safe.
- Some settings may be able to provide meals, or you may prefer to send your child with a packed lunch.
- Ongoing communication is key – keep reminding staff about your child's allergies, keep asking questions, be as involved as you can.

REFERENCES AND LINKS

- FPIES UK, 'Nursery & School' (n.d.)
  https://www.fpiesuk.org/for-parents/nursery-school/,
  accessed 13th March 2018.
- Muraro A, Clark A, Beyer K, Borrego LM, Borres M,
  Lødrup Carlsen KC, Carrer P, Mazon A, Rancè F,
  Valovirta E, Wickman M, Zanchetti M., 'The management
  of the allergic child at school: EEACI/GA2LEN Task
  Force on the allergic child at school', *Allergy*, 65 (2010),
  doi: 10.1111/j.1398-9995.2010.02343.x

CHAPTER 9

FAMILY AND FRIENDS

As a parent of a child with food allergies, you will sometimes need to enlist the help of others. Family and friends can be an important source of support. If people are willing to make the effort to make adaptations for your child, this can actually strengthen relationships and build trust. Unfortunately, family dynamics aren't always easy, and having a child with food allergies can sometimes be an extra source of tension. People don't always understand food allergies or may not realise how to accommodate your child's needs. Frequent communication is key to maintaining those family bonds whilst keeping your child safe and healthy.

You might experience problems such as:

- Not believing that food allergies are real, or not taking them seriously.
- Accidentally giving your child a food they are allergic to because they forgot to check the label.
- Giving them a food they are allergic to on purpose or even secretly, to try and prove that they are not really allergic to it, or to try and build up their tolerance.
- Thoughtlessly serving up foods at a family dinner that your child is allergic to.
- Constantly having to ask your relatives whether food

contains certain ingredients that your child is allergic to.

- Assuming that you are overreacting, neurotic or a control freak.

The reason for all these difficulties is that food allergies are invisible. Your child looks and behaves like any other child – unless they come into contact with a food they are allergic to. If your relatives haven't seen a reaction, they can find it difficult to accept. Think about your own attitudes to food allergies before you had your child – did you really understand what it was like?

Another reason why some people find it difficult to understand food allergies is because they are such a new issue. When we were growing up, food allergies were extremely rare. It's only recently that there has been a huge rise in the number of children with food allergies. Many older people don't have any previous experience of dealing with food allergies, and may need time to understand what it means for your child. Try and put yourself in their shoes and be patient if it takes them some time to really get it. Remember that they love your child and would never intentionally hurt them. Most people don't truly understand what it is like to have food allergies, but they want to.

COMMUNICATION

Family members should treat your child's food allergies with respect. They need to respect the physical aspects of keeping your child away from their allergen(s) and also the emotional impact of being different. Give them all the information they need in order to do this:

- Exactly which food(s) your child is allergic to.
- Signs and symptoms of a reaction.
- What to do in an emergency.
- What medication to give.

Explain that you are following the advice of your child's doctor by avoiding the food strictly to prevent a reaction, and that it is a not a lifestyle choice or fad.

You have a huge amount of experience and knowledge about your child's allergies – make sure you share this with relatives. It might help to show them some pages from this book, such as information on reading food labels (Chapter 4), how to avoid cross contact (Chapter 5), and food allergy myths (Chapter 14). Give them written information that they can keep and refer to, as they may not want to keep bothering you if they forget. Alternatively, get them to watch a video about food allergies (try Allergy Adventures on YouTube), and ideally watch it with them so you can discuss it.

Family members may feel sad about the changes that have to be made to accommodate your child's food allergies. For example, having to plan food in advance, not being able to cook a favourite recipe for a family gathering, etc. They may feel a sense of loss if get-togethers are not the same as they have been in the past, or what they had expected. Emphasise that these times are not just about food but about being together. They may also feel scared or anxious about accidentally causing your child to have a reaction.

Food can also be a way people show love and affection. If relatives want to give your child a treat, be strict about your food rules, but try to be flexible in other areas. You can suggest some alternative non-food 'treats' such as:

- staying up late
- taking your child to the park, zoo or other favourite place
- giving them a new toy, book, clothes or other gifts
- watching a movie together
- doing a craft or science experiment together.

If well-meaning relatives keep insisting that giving your child a little bit of the food they allergic to won't hurt, or that it might even help them to build up their immune system, you could ask your doctor to write a letter explaining that the current treatment for food allergies is strict avoidance.

Make it clear that when you double check food ingredients or food labels that it doesn't mean you don't trust them, it's just part of your routine as a food allergy parent. It's not their responsibility to be experts in food allergies, that's your responsibility as the parent until your child is old enough to do it themselves. Be understanding. If someone makes a mistake – and we are all only human after all – forgive, learn from it and move on.

FAMILY GATHERINGS

Most social events involve food, and children with food allergies can often end up feeling left out. It's always better for their emotional wellbeing if they can have the same food as everyone else whenever possible. Take responsibility for making sure your child is included. For example, if you are going out for a family meal, you can help to choose a suitable restaurant that you know will be safe for your child. For parties or informal get togethers, you can offer to bring food to share. Offer to host whenever you can.

Ask to check the labels of any food people want to give your child. Teach your children to always check with you first before accepting food from someone else. However, don't talk about food allergies all the time in front of your child as they just want to feel normal.

Another strategy is to suggest meetups that do not revolve around food e.g. meeting at the park, the zoo, going to the cinema, trips to the beach, going for a walk, and play dates (avoiding mealtimes).

Of course, you can't always organise every event. If there is a high-risk of cross contamination and you are unsure if the food is safe, bring your own food for your child. This might be appropriate for buffets, and also if your child's allergy is a common part of other people's diets, or if your child is newly diagnosed. Turn down invitations if they are too risky, but be gracious – not everything is about your child.

However, if you are finding that you have to pack food for your child at every social occasion, you need to consider whether your relatives are making enough of an effort to include your child as part of the family. They should at least try to provide some food that is safe, or choose a venue that can.

SETTING BOUNDARIES

Sometimes, people are unwilling or unable to be flexible, and you will have to stand up for your child. If this means refusing invitations to family gatherings, then so be it. Explain the emotional impact on your child, times when they have felt left out or gone hungry. For example, if they insist on eating Chinese food when your child is allergic to soya, this is unreasonable. They can always eat Chinese food another day. While your child is there, your relatives should choose something that means they can be included too. If your child had a visible disability and was in a wheelchair for example, your family would make adjustments. Someone else's desire for a particular food is not more important than your child's health and wellbeing.

On the other hand, your relatives may be unwilling to cook for your child because they don't understand which foods are safe and are afraid of accidentally making your child ill. Show them how to check food labels, wash hands and clean the kitchen and tools properly to avoid cross-contact. Reassure them that these small steps are extremely effective in preventing an allergic reaction.

It's really important to keep talking, and not just avoid your family, if this is the situation you find yourself in. You must explain directly, carefully and calmly why you are not going to social events. Your family members only need to take simple steps like reading and keeping food labels to keep your child safe. Be very clear about exactly what your child's needs are. An effective approach is to ask your relatives for help, rather than being demanding. Keep a positive attitude and suggest solutions rather than just complaining.

If they really don't get it and refuse to change, you will have to accept the situation and decide whether to continue your relationship with them in the same way.

Having a child with food allergies has an impact on the wider family as well as your life at home. Good communication is really important to make sure everyone knows how to keep your child safe. Teach your relatives what to do to minimise the risk of a reaction, whilst at the same time including your child in social gatherings as much as possible. The whole family will need to adapt, just as they would for any other medical condition or disability.

FRIENDSHIPS

Having food allergies can affect a child's friendships – both positively and negatively. If your child's friends learn about their allergies they can help look out for them and stick up for them in food-related situations. Good friends will want to help your child and make sure they can safely join in.

Allergy bullying can also be a problem. Most children with allergies are not bullied, but sadly some are. Young children may not understand the seriousness of food allergy, because they won't have seen someone having an allergic reaction. Having food allergies does make your child stand out from others and bullies will often pick on those children who are different. They may also be jealous if they feel your child is getting special attention because of their allergies.

For young children, bullying may come in the form of simple teasing, or saying things like "You're not allowed to come to my party because you can't eat the food." This can be hurtful and upsetting. Talk to the child's parents or your child's school about it.

In extreme cases other children may wave your child's food allergen in their face, attempt to put it on their skin or force them to eat it. This type of behaviour is potentially dangerous and must be tackled swiftly. It can cause physical harm and also increase anxiety for the child if they are afraid of the bully. Children who are scared of bullying may take more risks to try and fit in with their peers, such as not carrying their epinephrine auto-injectors or knowingly eating foods that might be unsafe.

Allergy bullying can be overcome with education about food allergies. In a school situation this can be best tackled by teaching all the children about food allergies and not just the bully.

Generally improving inclusiveness within the whole school helps to reduce bullying.

You can help prepare your child by talking about bullying in general. Make sure your child knows what bullying is and what to do if it happens to them (or one of their friends). Teach them how to stand up to bullies by saying "Stop!" or "Leave me alone" in a confident voice, or by walking away.

Ensure you know what the signs of bullying are – for food allergy kids this can include unexplained allergic reactions. Give plenty of opportunities for your child to talk to you about their school day. If they suddenly seem reluctant to go to school or change who they sit with at lunchtime, this can be a sign of a bullying problem. Of course, there could be other causes, but further investigation is needed.

BIRTHDAY PARTIES

Birthday parties are an important part of a child's social life. How you approach them will depend on the type and location of the party, how well you know the parents, and the severity of your child's allergies.

For parties at a commercial location such as a soft play or bowling alley, many venues will be able to cater for food allergies. Alternatively, if they are not able to provide suitable food they should allow your child to bring their own food to the party. Contact the venue yourself to make arrangements.

For parties in a village hall or at home where the parents are catering themselves, you will need to speak directly to them. If they are close friends they may be willing to adapt the party food to make it safe for your child. You can help them by telling them which brands of food to buy and which to avoid. You can tell them which sweets are safe to include for games like pass the parcel and in party bags.

Party food is often served buffet style which is a high risk for cross contact. Ask if your child can go to the buffet to take their food first, or have a plate of food pre-prepared and put aside for them. You can also offer to bring allergy friendly food to the party so that your child can at least eat one thing the same as every else e.g. a plate of cupcakes or rice crispie treats. If necessary, ask for the other children at the party to wash or wipe their hands after eating to keep your child safe.

Otherwise you will just need to let the host parents know that your child has allergies and will be bringing their own food. You may want to find out what type of food is being served at the party so you can provide similar food, e.g. dairy free pizza or ice cream. Ask if they can have a party plate to serve their food on so they don't feel too different.

If your child has severe food allergies you may want to ask to stay. If your child has an epinephrine auto-injector and you are dropping them off at the party you must explain to the hosts about your child's allergies, signs of a reaction, and what to do in an emergency. Give them a typed-up emergency plan they can refer to. However, you must have a good level of trust with the parents and if in any doubt just stay with your child at the party.

Alternatively (perhaps for an older child), you could drop your child off and wait nearby e.g. in the car or in a coffee shop. This may be difficult for you, but it will be empowering for your child to have independence. Ultimately, they do need to learn how to handle their allergies on their own. Teach your child how to politely decline food if it's offered.

If your child is unable to eat the birthday cake, it's a good idea to provide an alternative treat so they don't feel too left out. An easy way to do this is to bake a batch of suitable cupcakes, so that you can defrost one at a time as needed. Or you can bring a special treat that they don't normally have at home – as long as it feels like a special occasion.

Prepare your child for the party. Make sure they know whether they are allowed to eat the party food or if they should only eat food from their lunchbox. Reassure them that they will have lots of tasty food! Explain which adults at the party know about the food allergy. Make sure your child's feels confident so that when they are at the party they can focus on having fun without worrying about food.

Sometimes your child might not be invited to a party due to their allergies. In this case you may want to talk to the parents. They may not understand how to include your child. In rare cases it may not be safe for your child under any circumstances e.g. a birthday party at an ice cream parlour if your child has a severe milk allergy.

Managing relationships and social events can be challenging as a parent of a child with food allergies. Once again it takes a higher level of organisation. Ongoing communication is really key. It can also be stressful for you as you are not in control and your child's food allergen might be present. However, when you overcome these challenges, your child can still enjoy a normal social life.

KEY POINTS

- It may take time for friends and family members to get used to the idea that your child has food allergies.
- Family gatherings and birthday parties will need consideration of how to avoid your child's food allergen(s).
- Some children are bullied because of food allergies – be aware of the signs.
- Friends and family can become a great source of help and support for children with food allergies.

REFERENCES AND LINKS

- Black, M. Carolyn, 'Caution, Relatives Ahead', *Allergic Living* (July 2010), https://www.allergicliving.com/2010/07/02/food-allergy-caution-relatives-ahead/, accessed 25th February 2018.
- Black, M. Carolyn, 'Family Food Feud: Relatives and Allergies', *Allergic Living* (December 2010), https://www.allergicliving.com/2010/12/07/family-food-feud/, accessed 25th February 2018.
- Clowes, Gina, '7 Ways to Resolve Food Allergy Issues with

Family and Friends', *Allergic Living* (November 2016), https://www.allergicliving.com/2016/11/14/7-ways-resolve-food-allergy-issues-family-friends/, accessed 25th February 2018.

- Food Allergy & Anaphylaxis Connection Team, 'Bullying Resources for Educators and Parents' (n.d.), https://www.foodallergyawareness.org/education/bullying/bullying-resources/, accessed 25th February 2018.

- Food Allergy Research & Education, 'Bullying Prevention: What You Can Do' (n.d.), https://www.foodallergy.org/life-with-food-allergies/living-well-everyday/bullying-prevention/what-you-can-do, accessed 25th February 2018.

- French, Janet, 'Food Allergy Bullying: How to Spot if Your Child is a Target and Actions to Take', *Allergic Living* (May 2018), https://www.allergicliving.com/2018/05/15/food-allergy-bullying-how-to-spot-if-your-child-is-a-target-and-actions-to-take/, accessed 25th February 2018.

- Lester, Stephanie, 'Relatives Who Don't 'Get' Food Allergies', *Allergic Living* (December 2010), https://www.allergicliving.com/2010/12/08/relatives-who-dont-get-food-allergies/2/, accessed 25th February 2018.

- Smartt, Jessica, 'How To Love A Family With Food Allergies' [blog], *The Humbled Homemaker* (April 2015), https://thehumbledhomemaker.com/love-family-food-allergies/, accessed 25th February 2018.

- Smartt, Jessica, 'What Parents Of Kids With Food Allergies Want You To Know (But Are Afraid To Say)' [blog], *Smartter Each Day* (February 2014), http://smarttereachday.com/what-parents-of-kids-with-allergies-wish-you-knew-but-are-afraid-to-tell-you/, accessed 25th February 2018.

- Smith, Nicole, 'Emotional Aspects Of Food Allergies And Extended Family', *Allergic Child* (November 2011), http://home.allergicchild.com/emotional-aspects-of-food-allergies-and-extended-family/, accessed 25th February 2018.

- Studer Daley, Jennifer, 'Tips For Educating Your Friends

And Family About Food Allergies', *Food Allergy Research &
Education* (June 2017), https://www.foodallergy.org/about-
fare/blog/tips-for-educating-your-friends-and-family-
about-food-allergies, accessed 25th February 2018.

CHAPTER 10

GROWING OUT OF ALLERGIES

Growing out of food allergies is known in medical terms as 'achieving tolerance'. More than a quarter of children do grow out of their food allergies, usually by the age of 5. It is thought this may be due to the gut maturing or changes in the immune system response. Children are highly likely to grow out of allergies to eggs, milk, wheat and soya. Unfortunately, children with allergies to peanuts, seafood, fish, and tree nuts only rarely grow out of their allergies, and if they do it can take longer, usually by age 10 or 12. The earlier your child had their first allergic reaction, the more likely they are to outgrow their allergy.

Your child has a better chance of outgrowing their food allergy if they only have mild to moderate symptoms, are allergic to only one food, or have eczema as their only symptom. Children with severe symptoms such as anaphylaxis or those with multiple food allergies are much less likely to grow out of their allergies.

IN HOSPITAL OR AT HOME?

A food challenge is when you deliberately give your child a food they have previously reacted to, to see if they have grown out of their allergy. If your child has ever had severe reactions such as wheezing, throat tightening or floppiness (anaphylaxis) you should never try a food challenge at home. You should only attempt a food challenge as advised by a health professional, under medical supervision in a hospital or allergy clinic.

If your child has only mild or moderate reactions, or has delayed reactions, your health professional may advise you to try a food challenge at home. You will introduce the food in a controlled way, starting with a very small amount and building up the amount of food given very gradually.

PICKING THE RIGHT TIME

You should wait at least 6-12 months from your child's last allergic reaction before starting a new food challenge (or longer if your health professional advises it). Only start when your child is well, with no colds or tummy upsets, and not teething. Your child's skin should be clear with no eczema flare-ups. If they have asthma this should be well controlled as well.

Home life should be settled, so avoid starting a food challenge at the same time as any big changes such as starting nursery or school, potty training or moving house for example. Although stress does not cause allergies, it can make allergic reactions worse. Don't start a food challenge just before a special occasion such a birthday or a holiday, because if your child does have a reaction you don't want them to be unwell and miss out on the fun.

If your child is starting any new medication, wait at least two weeks until your child is settled on the medication before starting a food challenge.

If your child takes regular antihistamines e.g. for hayfever or other seasonal allergies, these medicines will mask an allergic reaction. They will either need to stop taking the medication, find alternative medication or wait until the seasons change. Ask your health professional for advice on how to do this. Any other regular medication should be taken as prescribed.

You should also have enough time during the day to do the food challenge and monitor your child afterwards, for example on a quiet day at home. This is especially important if your child has immediate reactions.

If there is any doubt about whether it is the right time to do the food challenge, it is best to wait until you feel certain. You may have to wait several weeks or months to find a good time – be patient and don't rush.

PREPARING YOUR CHILD FOR THE FOOD CHALLENGE

Food challenge in hospital

Your child's doctor will only suggest a food challenge if their skin prick or blood tests are negative and they have a good chance of reintroducing the food successfully, depending on their history. The food is only introduced gradually, starting with tiny amounts, to reduce the risk of a severe reaction.

If you are doing a food challenge in hospital you will need to think about how you will talk to your child about it, depending on their age and level of understanding. Be honest with them, stay calm, be positive and use age-appropriate language. For example, you could explain that the doctor thinks they may have grown out of their allergy, but to know for sure you have to try eating the food. They will have medicine at the hospital just in case the food does make them feel poorly. If they have grown out of their allergy, they would be able to eat the same food as their friends.

For a younger child you can prepare them with role play and act out with toys or puppets what will happen at the hospital. When you arrive, your child will have their temperature, pulse and blood pressure taken, and this will be repeated throughout the day. Then they will be given a small amount of their food allergen to eat. They will be monitored for a reaction and then, if they are fine, they will be given increasing amounts of food, until a full dose is reached.

An older child might feel scared or worried about eating some of the food that they have been taught to avoid. Don't brush fears aside or just tell your child "you'll be fine". Give them the chance to ask questions and talk about their worries so you can address them. If they seem upset, you can ask them, "What are you worried about?" and then just listen. Encourage them to be specific about their fears, so that together you can find a way deal with it. This will also help your child feel more willing to go along with the food challenge.

Reassure your child that it is safe to do a hospital food challenge. It is done with experienced doctors and nurses there who are used to looking after children with food allergies. They will have all the necessary medicines and equipment on hand, just in case your child does have a reaction. You will be with your child the whole time.

Depending on your child's allergy you may be asked to bring some food containing your child's allergen with you for the food challenge. For example, if your child has egg allergy you may be asked to make some muffins containing egg and bring them with you. You might also be asked to bring a food that your child normally eats, that their allergen can be hidden in. For example, ground nuts can be stirred into yogurt.

Bring things for you and your child to do at the hospital, as you may need to be there for several hours, or even a whole day. For example, colouring books, stickers, reading books, board games or toys. Maybe buy them something new that they haven't seen before, as that will hold their attention for longer. If they have a favourite soft toy or blanket that they use for comfort, bring that. You will also need to bring safe food to eat while you are waiting.

Plan for the food challenge to take up the whole day – don't make plans afterwards, as even if it goes well it will be stressful and draining for both of you. If you have other children, arrange for someone else to look after them that day.

Be prepared that your child may refuse to eat the food, perhaps if they are feeling very nervous or if they don't like the taste of it. You and the hospital staff can encourage your child to eat the food, but the hospital will not force them to eat it. In this case the challenge will be rescheduled for another day.

HOSPITAL FOOD CHALLENGE: WHAT ARE THE RISKS?

A 2015 study, which reviewed food challenges completed for wheat, soy, milk, egg, peanut, seeds, tree nuts, fish, shellfish and other foods over a 10-year period at The Children's Hospital of Philadelphia, found that 70% of hospital food challenges are successful. Wheat and soy had the lowest rate of reactions, with milk, peanut and egg the highest.

An older study, published in 2004, found that of 584 food challenges, 43% resulted in an allergic reaction, but no children were hospitalised and there were no deaths. Again, milk, egg and peanut challenges were most likely to have a reaction. Wheat and soy challenges were least likely to have a reaction. Children with eczema, asthma, allergic rhinitis or multiple food allergies were more likely to have a reaction. Of the 253 children who did have a reaction, 72% had a mild to moderate reaction and 28% had a severe reaction (71 children).

A further study from 2012, showed that very few reactions happened at the first 'dose' of the food allergen and most reactions happened after the maximum dose. A small proportion of children who had a reaction did experience anaphylaxis. Again, there were no deaths.

Gupta, Malika et al. "Egg Food Challenges Are Associated with More Gastrointestinal Reactions." Ed. Sari Acra. *Children* 2.3 (2015): 371–381
https://dx.doi.org/10.3390%2Fchildren2030371
Perry TT, Matsui EC, Conover-Walker MK, Wood RA. "Risk of oral food challenges." *Journal of Allergy and Clinical Immunology* 2004 114(5):1164-8
http://www.jacionline.org/article/S0091-6749(04)02289-4/fulltext
Rolinck-Werninghaus C, Niggemann B, Grabenhenrich L, Wahn U and Beyer K. "Outcome of oral food challenges in children in relation to symptom-eliciting allergen dose and allergen-specific IgE." Abstract. *Allergy* 2012 67(7):951-7
https://www.ncbi.nlm.nih.gov/pubmed/22583105/

Food challenge at home

For a home food challenge, you have the choice whether to tell your child about the challenge or not. It depends on your preference, how old your child is, and their temperament. It also depends on how easily you can hide the fact that you are doing the food challenge!

Before starting the food challenge, make sure you have children's antihistamine in the house, which you can give your child if they have a reaction. Review the signs and symptoms of a reaction so you know what to look out for (see overleaf). Only introduce one new food at a time. Continue to avoid any other foods that your child is allergic or intolerant to.

For milk, egg, wheat and soya allergies, you will follow a 'ladder' to reintroduce the food gradually at home. Your dietitian will provide you with a ladder for your child. Different trusts within the NHS have developed their own ladders and so there is some variation depending on where you live. Some examples of these are given later in this chapter.

STARTING THE LADDER

If your child is very sensitive, but you have been advised to do a food challenge at home, follow the advice below. If your child has mild/moderate or delayed reactions, you may be able to skip this step and just start by eating the food. If in doubt, it is better to go slower. This advice is here as general guidance.

1. If your child has had a previous reaction on skin contact with the food, start by rubbing a small amount of the food on your child's cheek or inner arm.
2. Wait for around 30 minutes to see if there is a reaction, allowing your child to carry on with their normal activities.
3. If there are no signs of a reaction, you can rub a small amount of the food on the inside of your child's lips.
4. Wait for 30 minutes to see if there is a reaction.
5. If there is still no reaction you can give them a crumb of food to eat.

Immediate reactions usually happen within a couple of hours, delayed reactions can be hours or even a day or two later. For a reminder of the symptoms to look out for see overleaf. If your child has a reaction at any stage, stop the food challenge and give them any medication if necessary. Continue to monitor them for 6-10 hours as once an allergic reaction has started, some symptoms can develop later.

If your child has a severe reaction you should contact your doctor once they are feeling better and ask for reassessment of their allergy management.

MOVING UP THE LADDER

If your child doesn't have a reaction you can gradually increase the amount of the food, roughly doubling the amount of food every 1-3 days (a crumb first, then a pea-sized amount, then a teaspoonful and so on). Keep increasing the amount of food until they are eating a normal child-sized portion. Make sure you give them the food every day to build their tolerance. You may need to spend anywhere from one week to several weeks on each step of the ladder, so allow plenty of time and don't rush.

Once your child is regularly eating the first food without any symptoms, you can move onto the next step. If at any stage your child shows a mild/moderate reaction to the food, go back to the previous step on the ladder. Keep giving them the food from that step of the ladder, and any previous steps, regularly (at least 2-3 times a week). This will maintain their level of tolerance. Do not go back to the beginning or stop altogether. Try the next step again in 6 months' time, or as advised by your health professional.

Keep a diary of exactly which foods you are introducing and what portion size your child has eaten, along with any suspected symptoms. This can help you to keep track of how much of the food your child can tolerate. It's also helpful for mild or delayed reactions as symptoms may build up over a few days or a week. If you fail at any step of the ladder this diary can help you to work out what amount of food your child can tolerate until you can try to move up the ladder again.

MILD TO MODERATE SYMPTOMS

Give antihistamines and/or asthma medication if needed.

- Tingly or itchy mouth
- Feeling very hot or very cold
- Itchy skin
- Rash appearing on the skin (hives)
- Swelling, especially on the face
- Feeling scared or anxious
- Feeling or being sick
- Stomach pains
- Pale skin
- Mild wheeziness

SEVERE SYMPTOMS – CALL 999 AND ASK FOR AN AMBULANCE

- Difficulty breathing e.g. wheezing, hoarseness or croupy cough
- Feeling faint
- Becoming pale and floppy
- Collapse

DELAYED REACTIONS (USUALLY AFTER 2 HOURS AND WITHIN 3 DAYS)

- Loose and/or frequent stools
- Stomach pains
- Constipation
- Blood and/or mucus in stools
- Reflux and/or heartburn
- Eczema

Note that slightly softer/harder stools are not a cause for concern on their own.

If the food you are trying is tolerated, you should continue to give them the food regularly, as well as all the foods on the previous steps – at least 2-3 times a week. If you stop giving them the food for a long period of time, they can lose their tolerance and the allergy may return.

Some children might grow to tolerate their food allergen, but if they eat more than a certain amount they start to have allergic symptoms. For example, one glass of cow's milk a day, two slices of bread a day, one boiled egg a day. If this is the case then keep giving your child the amount that they can tolerate.

Be aware that your child might not want to eat the food you are giving them. For example, if they are not used to eating egg they might not like the taste or texture. Keep offering it but don't force them to eat it. You can try eating the food in front of them and just ask them if they would like to try a little bit. Seeing you eating the food can help them accept it. Alternatively, you may need to hide the foods in something they are used to eating. For example you could hide a teaspoon of grated cheese inside a tuna sandwich, or a teaspoon of wheat flour mixed into a yogurt. You may need to experiment with different foods on the same step of the ladder, if possible. If your child is refusing to eat the food and you are unable to do the food challenge at all, ask your health professional for advice.

MILK LADDER

Below is a guide to the full iMAP 12-step milk ladder. There are shorter versions available – always follow the version your dietitian gives you. For recipes with full instructions to go with the milk ladder, see the 'References and Links' section at the end of this chapter. At each step guidance is given of what size portion to give your child.

Step 1: Malted milk biscuits
- If using shop bought, choose biscuits that contain milk powder and not whey powder in the ingredients
- Start with 1 biscuit
- If tolerated, increase to 2 biscuits

Step 2: Garibaldi biscuits/digestives
- If using shop bought, choose biscuits that contain milk
- Start with half a biscuit
- If tolerated, increase to 1 biscuit

Step 3: Mini muffins/cupcakes
- Start with half a muffin or cake (15g)
- If tolerated, increase to 1 muffin/cake (30g)

Step 4: Scotch pancakes
- If using shop bought, choose ones that contain milk powder and not whey powder in the ingredients
- Start with 1 scotch pancake
- If tolerated, increase to 3 scotch pancakes

Step 5: Shepherd's Pie
- Make sure the mash topping contains milk and/or butter
- Give 200g shepherd's pie
- If tolerated, move onto the next step

Step 6: Lasagne
- Give 200g lasagne
- If tolerated, move onto the next step

Step 7: Pizza
- Start with half a mini pizza
- If tolerated, increase to 1 whole mini pizza

Step 8: Milk chocolate
- Start with 10g chocolate or chocolate buttons
- If tolerated, increase to 35g

Step 9: Yogurt
- Give 1 pot yogurt
- If tolerated, move onto the next step

Step 10: Cheese
- Give 25g hard cheese such as cheddar

Step 11: Sterilised milk/infant formula (in cartons) – often labelled as long life/UHT milk and does not need to be kept in the fridge until you open the carton.

- Start with 100ml
- If tolerated, increase to 200ml

Step 12: Pasteurised fresh milk/powdered infant formula
- Start with 100ml
- If tolerated, increase to 200ml.

ALTERNATIVE FOODS

If you have to stop part way through the milk ladder, your child will still benefit from being able to eat more different types of foods. While you are waiting to move up the milk ladder, you can try introducing some of the other foods suggested below. If your child won't eat the main food suggested on the milk ladder, you can try these alternatives instead.

If your child can tolerate **digestive/garibaldi biscuit** they can also try other biscuits containing milk.

If your child can tolerate **cakes/muffins and scotch pancakes** they can also try waffles, pastry, shortbread, croissant, plain brioche, flatbreads containing milk/yogurt as an ingredient, breakfast cereals containing added milk, frozen Yorkshire puddings, shop bought pancakes, processed meats containing milk (e.g. frankfurters, pate), cheesy breadsticks, crackers or biscuits and flavourings that contain milk e.g. crisps. At this stage they may also be able to tolerate butter.

If your child can tolerate **shepherd's pie** they can also try other types of pie with mashed potato topping containing milk and butter such as fish pie, chicken pie or hotpot with mash topping, and also potato croquettes.

If your child can tolerate **lasagne** they can also try other foods containing dairy that are baked for 30 minutes such as pasta bakes, baked fish, baked macaroni cheese, cauliflower cheese, oven baked rice pudding, and oven baked bread and butter pudding.

If your child can tolerate **pizza** they can also try cheese on toast, custard, custard tart, rice pudding, cheese sauce, white sauce, cream soups, homemade pancakes and Yorkshire puddings.

If your child can tolerate **yogurt** they can also try fromage frais, yogurt drinks and soft cheese e.g. cream cheese, camembert, brie.

If your child can tolerate **hard cheese** e.g. cheddar they can also try uncooked milk desserts such as ice cream (one small scoop).

EGG LADDER

Step 1: Well-cooked egg
- Cakes
- Biscuits
- Dried egg pasta
- Egg in sausages and vegetarian sausages
- Egg in processed meat products such as burgers and meatballs
- Well-cooked fresh egg pasta
- Quorn
- Sponges and sponge fingers
- Dried egg noodles
- Cakes
- Biscuits containing egg e.g. gingerbread
- Waffles
- Chocolate containing nougat or dried egg e.g. Milky Way, Mars Bar, Crème Egg
- Sweets containing egg e.g. Chewits
- Pancakes and Yorkshire pudding – if well cooked and not soggy

Step 2: Lightly cooked egg
- Pancakes
- Yorkshire pudding
- Scrambled, boiled, poached or fried egg
- Omelette
- Egg fried rice

- Meringue
- Marshmallows containing egg
- Lemon curd
- Quiche
- Egg in batter e.g. some battered fish
- Egg in breadcrumbs e.g. some fish fingers or chicken nuggets
- Hollandaise sauce
- Flans
- Egg custard and egg custard tarts
- Crème caramel
- Fresh custard (not instant)
- Tempura batter

Step 3: Foods containing raw egg
- Mayonnaise
- Fresh mousse containing egg
- Fresh ice cream containing egg
- Sorbet containing egg
- Royal icing
- Home-made marzipan
- Raw egg in cake mix and mixes (licking the spoon)
- Egg glaze on pastry
- Horseradish sauce
- Tartar sauce
- Salad cream

WHEAT LADDER

For steps 1 and 2, start with a small piece of food or ¼ spoonful for the first two or three days, then increase gradually.

Step 1: Foods containing a small amount of wheat, for example:
- stock cubes
- gravy
- sauces
- pâté

- soups
- processed meats
- sausages

Step 2: Foods with wheat as the main ingredient:
For example: wheat-based breakfast cereal, pasta, bread, biscuits, cakes etc.

Step 3: Eating wheat regularly:
Continue to increase the amount of wheat your child is eating, until they are eating wheat freely.

SOYA LADDER

Step 1: Soya lecithin (skip this step if already tolerating soya lecithin)
- Foods containing soya lecithin as an ingredient (found in many processed foods and chocolate) – eat one normal child-size portion e.g. 1 bag chocolate buttons. If you know your child is very sensitive to soya lecithin, start with a smaller portion.

Step 2: Baked food containing soya – choose one of the following:
- Bread containing soya flour – start with ½ slice bread and build up to 1 slice bread
- Biscuits or cakes containing soya – start with 1 biscuit and build up to 2 biscuits

Step 3: Whole soya food – choose one of the following:
- Soya yogurt, dessert or custard – start with 2 heaped teaspoons and double the amount each day, building up to 125g (1 pot)
- Homemade soya custard using Bird's custard powder and soya milk – start with 2 heaped teaspoons and build up to 125g

Step 4: Soya milk
- Start with 50ml soya milk and increase by 50ml each day, until your child is drinking their usual milk volume.

Step 5: Continue to increase the amount of soya your child is eating, until they are eating soya freely.

HOW TO CONSTRUCT YOUR OWN FOOD LADDER FOR OTHER ALLERGIES

If your child has a more unusual food allergy you will need to make up your own food ladder. Cooked or processed versions of a food are usually more easily tolerated. Look for foods that contain the allergen as an ingredient further down the ingredients list to begin with. For example, if your child is allergic to oats you could start with multigrain cereal, sausages containing oats, or bread containing oats, before moving on to foods like flapjacks and porridge which have oats as a main ingredient. For legumes, you might start with sausages or bread containing pea protein (often found in gluten free foods), then try poppadoms before attempting whole peas or beans. If you are not sure, speak to a dietitian for advice.

Reintroducing a food to your child's diet that you have been avoiding for a long time can feel nerve-wracking. Take it slowly and don't rush yourself. With luck, your child will have grown out of their allergy and they will be able to eat the food again. It can be disappointing if they have a reaction at any stage, but focus on the progress you have made, even if it is just to learn more about how they react to the food. Good luck!

KEY POINTS

- Some children will grow out of their food allergy and be able to eat the food they were once allergic to, or have partial tolerance to it.
- Giving your child a food they are allergic to, to see if they have grown out of their allergy, is called a food challenge.
- For severe allergies, food challenges are done in hospital.
- For mild or moderate allergies, food challenges can be done at home.
- Foods are reintroduced gradually, starting with a small amount and building up slowly.

REFERENCES AND LINKS

- Food Allergy Research & Education, 'Who Is Likely to Outgrow A Food Allergy?' (September 2013), https://www.foodallergy.org/about-fare/blog/who-is-likely-to-outgrow-a-food-allergy, accessed 11th December 2018.

- Gupta, RS Lau, CH Sita, EE Smith, BB and Greenhawt, MJ, 'Factors associated with reported food allergy tolerance among US children', *Annals of Allergy, Asthma & Immunology*, 111, 3 (2013), doi: 10.1016/j.anai.2013.06.026.

- Robertson, Clare and Ward , Judith, 'How to do an egg and cow's milk challenge at home' *Oxford University Hospitals NHS Trust* (July 2013), https://www.ouh.nhs.uk/patient-guide/leaflets/files/5538Peggmilkchallenge.pdf, accessed 11th December 2018.

- Venter, C, Brown, T, Shah, N, Walsh, J, Fox AT, 'The Milk Ladder', *The MAP Guideline* (October 2013), http://ifan.ie/wp-content/uploads/2014/02/Milk-Ladder-2013-MAP.pdf, accessed 11th December 2018.

- Venter, C, Barnard, P, Brady, I, Denton, SA, Carling, A, Greenland, C, Heather, N, Weeks, R, Lajeunesse, M, 'Recipes to go with MAP Milk Ladder' (April 2013) http://ifan.ie/wp-content/uploads/2015/10/MAP-Milk-Ladder-Additional-Recipes-Oct-2015.pdf, accessed 11th December 2018.

CHAPTER 11

THE FUTURE OF FOOD ALLERGIES

Food allergies have increased drastically in recent years, and are still increasing. By 2050, a whopping 45-50% of children in the UK are expected to suffer from food allergies. To understand why, scientists are studying the causes of food allergies, as well as how to prevent them, diagnosing food allergies and possible cures.

TRENDS IN FOOD ALLERGIES

The most common food allergies vary from country to country. Globally, cow's milk allergy is the most frequently diagnosed allergy. Reactions to milk are becoming more common, more severe, and more persistent. This means that more children are having severe reactions to milk than ever before. Fewer children are growing out of their milk allergy, and for those that do outgrow their milk allergy it is taking longer. It is becoming increasingly likely to remain allergic to milk even into adulthood.

A link has been found between food allergies, eczema and asthma. A child may appear to outgrow food allergies, but then later develop childhood eczema, and a few years after that show signs of asthma and hayfever. This is known as the 'allergic march'. Research is looking into tackling allergic diseases early in life to prevent this progression. As a result, new treatments for babies with food allergies may also help to stop them getting eczema, asthma or hayfever as they get older.

APPROACHES TO TREATING FOOD ALLERGIES

The traditional approach to managing food allergies is very passive. The only treatment is to completely avoid the problem food(s) and wait and hope that the child will outgrow the allergy. As the child gets older they may have repeat blood or skin prick tests and/or try food challenges to see if they have grown out of their allergy.

Now we are moving towards a more active model for treating food allergies. This includes introducing food allergens early in life to prevent allergies developing in the first place (see Chapter 3 for more on this). At the same time, strategies for increasing a person's tolerance are being developed such as Oral Immunotherapy, which is explained later in this chapter.

CAUSES OF FOOD ALLERGIES

The gut microbiome is a huge new area of research with regard to food allergy. Studies have found that infants with food allergies have different types of gut bacteria compared to those without. One particular type of good bacteria that is known to be a marker of a healthy gut microbiome is called bifidobacteria. Levels of this particular species of bacteria are lower in babies with food allergies. Babies with food allergies also have fewer different types of gut bacteria – more variety decreases the chances of having food allergies.

Factors that can affect a baby's gut bacteria include:
- How the baby was born (C-section or vaginal birth)
- How many weeks into pregnancy the baby was born
- Infections
- Feeding patterns
- Antibiotics
- Genetics
- Immune system
- Maternal factors

However, this research is still in its infancy and lots more still needs to be done. One focus for upcoming research is to find out the exact differences between the gut microbiome of a healthy child vs an allergic child. Scientists are also looking at which strains of probiotics can be used to treat allergies, what dose to use and for how long (more on this later in the chapter).

DIAGNOSING FOOD ALLERGIES

The current allergy tests available only work for IgE-mediated allergies (immediate reactions – see Chapter 1). These are currently diagnosed by a blood test which looks for IgE antibodies, or by a skin-prick test (or both). These tests are used both to diagnose food allergies and later to see if a patient has grown out of their allergy. However, the blood tests are not always accurate and results may come back positive even though the child is not actually allergic to the food being tested. This may mean that some patients are avoiding foods that they are not actually allergic to. Skin prick tests are also unreliable and can sometimes come back positive when a person can eat the food without having any symptoms, and vice versa.

Work is being done into improving the current IgE tests, by testing for many different IgE antibodies at the same time, and by breaking down foods into more specific allergens. This would be much more accurate and also help doctors to predict how severe a person's allergies are, using a small amount of blood from just one blood test.

At the moment there are no tests for non-IgE-mediated allergies, (delayed reactions – see Chapter 1). Currently these must be diagnosed by an exclusion diet. Patch testing is still used by some specialists but this is rare, because it is very difficult to perform the tests consistently. A focus for future research is to develop a test to improve diagnosis of non-IgE food allergies.

A new blood test is being developed which tests for MAST cells, which are another type of cells involved in allergic reactions. In a study, this was found to be much more accurate than the current tests used. They may even be suitable for both IgE- and non-IgE-mediated allergies. This would make it easier for doctors to accurately diagnose food allergies, reduce the number of people avoiding foods they are not actually allergic to, and make it easier to know when it is safe to reintroduce a food.

Another area of study is whether food allergies can be diagnosed by a urine test. Researchers have used new technology to discover a substance found in the urine called PGDM which is linked with food allergy. The amount of PGDM found relates to the severity of the allergy. This type of test is in the very early stages of development, but it would mean that food allergies could be diagnosed without needing a blood test. It is also a more sensitive test that can tell you how severe your allergy is. However, it cannot detect which food you are allergic to, and so additional tests may be needed alongside it.

TREATMENTS FOR FOOD ALLERGIES

Please note that these therapies are always conducted by allergy experts in a medical setting and are not safe to try at home as there is a risk of anaphylaxis.

Oral immunotherapy (OIT) build up a person's tolerance to a food by giving them increasing amounts of that food, starting with a very tiny dose and building up gradually over time. This approach has been researched and developed over the past 25 years. When it works, the person no longer has to avoid the food, and may even be able to eat it on a regular basis if they wish. Once the therapy is completed, there is a 'maintenance dose' of the food which has to be eaten daily to prevent the allergy from returning.

OIT has only been shown to work for IgE-mediated allergies (see Chapter 1 for more on different types of allergies). The therapy has been shown to be safe, although there is a very small risk of anaphylaxis in some patients. Most patients do experience some mild symptoms at first such as hives, itchy mouth or upset stomach, which then go away. This therapy is very successful at reducing a person's sensitivity to a food allergen. Because the therapy is quite new, it is too soon to tell if the benefits will stay over a longer period of time.

Oral immunotherapy is thought to be more successful the younger you do it. Promising research is also being done into whether success rates can be boosted by giving a probiotic at the same time. One study found that by combining OIT with a probiotic, the protection against allergies remains after a few years, even without a maintenance dose.

An alternative to this is to use a daily skin patch. This is known as Epicutaneous immunotherapy, or EPIT. This would provide protection from severe reactions to accidental exposure, but wouldn't allow a person to eat the food they were previously allergic to. You would still need to be careful about avoiding foods containing large amount of nuts, for example, but may not need to worry about foods labelled as 'may contains nuts' or cross contact from other people who have eaten nuts. EPIT could be a good treatment for people who have a bad reaction to oral immunotherapy, do not want to try it, or find it difficult to eat their food allergens every day.

These therapies are still undergoing clinical trials in the UK so it will be some time before they will be available on the NHS, although some specialist clinics are beginning to offer them privately. Researchers are still working out the exact methods they need to follow to have the highest chance of success.

PREBIOTICS, PROBIOTICS AND SYNBIOTICS

We saw earlier in the chapter that the gut microbiome has a huge role to play in allergic disease. Gut bacteria can be changed by using prebiotics, probiotics or synbiotics. However, this is best done early in life as the older you get, the harder it is to change your gut microbiome.

KEY TERMS

Probiotics: Live bacteria that are beneficial to the body.
Prebiotics: Substances that help good bacteria to grow – basically food for the probiotics.
Synbiotic: A combination of prebiotics and probiotics. Taking both together helps the probiotics to work better.

The best way to improve a baby's gut microbiome is breastfeeding. We have already covered breastfeeding in general terms in Chapter 3. Breastmilk already contains natural prebiotics and probiotics. Breastfed babies have better intestinal flora with higher proportions of good bacteria and fewer bad bacteria.

Scientists are beginning to develop baby formula milk with prebiotics/probiotics/synbiotics. Some recent studies have shown that this type of supplemented formula reduces the rate of allergic diseases such as food allergies, eczema and asthma. However, at this stage not enough is known about the best strains of bacteria to include, how much to include, and for how long.

If you would like to try giving your baby or child with food allergies probiotics, it is reassuring to know that they have been shown to do no harm. The only exception is in children who are immunocompromised. Look for brands that contain strains of Bifidobacterium and Lactobacilli, as these are known to be beneficial. Choose one that is specifically designed for your child's age, to ensure they get a suitable dose. If your child is allergic to cow's milk, check that the product is suitable, as some probiotics are grown in cow's milk.

Remember that you get what you pay for and cheap probiotics may not give you any benefit. It is worth spending more to get a higher quality, more effective probiotic.

There may be some symptoms when introducing probiotics such as an increase in wind or a change in your baby's poos. This is normal and should settle down. However, if you are concerned you can reduce the amount you are giving to your child and build up more gradually.

PREVENTING FOOD ALLERGIES

If you already have a child with food allergies and you are thinking about having more children in the future, you may be wondering if there's anything you can do to prevent your future children from developing allergies? The bad news is, that there is nothing that has been proven to completely *prevent* food allergies. The good news is that there are things you can do to *reduce* the chances of your baby developing food allergies.

PREGNANCY

You don't need to change your diet during pregnancy. Avoiding common allergens during pregnancy does not have any effect on your baby's chances of developing an allergy. Generally, you should aim to eat a healthy, balanced diet during pregnancy, with plenty of vegetables and fruit.

Taking fish oil omega-3 supplements during pregnancy can reduce the chances of your baby developing a food allergy. One study found that taking fish oil omega-3 supplements can cut the rate of egg allergy by almost a third, and may also reduce the chances of peanut allergy (other allergies haven't been studied yet). Choose supplements labelled as 'omega-3 fish oil'. Avoid supplements containing fish liver, such as cod liver oil. These contain high levels of vitamin A which can harm your baby. You can also get omega-3 from foods such as oily fish. Pregnant women should not eat more than two portions of oily fish a week.

Probiotics may help to reduce the likelihood of your baby developing cow's milk allergy and childhood eczema. There is not enough evidence yet to suggest which probiotics are best. Look for brands that can provide evidence of a benefit. Look at how many live bacteria are in the product. This may be listed as CFUs (colony forming units). Choose one that is in the billions.

Research suggests that folic acid supplements taken whilst pregnant may increase the risk of food allergies in the infant. However, the reason for this is not known. Folic acid supplements are recommended for all women whilst trying to conceive, and during pregnancy, as it helps prevent serious neural tube defects. To be able to use folic acid, the body must convert it to its natural form, folate. It may be that some people are less able to convert the folic acid in this way, and so it builds up in the body.

Your body needs folate during pregnancy to ensure the normal growth and development of your baby. You can get some folate from your diet, but the government recommends all pregnant women take supplements. Look for supplements containing folate instead of folic acid to get the benefits without the risk. This would be listed as 5-methyltetrahydrofolate" or "5-MTHF" on the label. If you are unsure, discuss this with a health professional.

BREASTFEEDING

There is some evidence to suggest that exclusively breastfeeding for the first six months may decrease your baby's chance of developing eczema, asthma and food allergy. You do not need to change your diet (apart from to avoid any allergens that you already know about, if they react to foods you have eaten). Continuing to take probiotics and fish oil while breastfeeding also helps to reduce the chances of developing allergic disease.

Food allergies will be a huge area of scientific interest in the next few years because it affects increasing numbers of people, and because it places a huge burden on medical services. There seems to be a new study on food allergies published every week or two. This should mean huge advances in our knowledge about food allergies as well as new treatments in the coming years.

KEY POINTS

- Scientists are still trying to understand why food allergies are on the rise. This is thought to have multiple causes.
- New, more accurate tests are being developed, as well as tests for non-IgE food allergies.
- Treatments that involve giving the child a very tiny amount of their food allergen to reduce the risk of a severe reaction are currently undergoing clinical trials.
- Probiotics are thought to have potential as a way of treating food allergies.
- Some supplements taken during pregnancy and/or breastfeeding may affect the chances of your baby developing food allergies.

REFERENCES AND LINKS

- American Academy of Allergy Asthma & Immunology, 'Folic Acid Exposure In Utero Is Associated With Development Of Food Allergy' (2018), https://www.aaaai.org/about-aaaai/newsroom/news-releases/folic-acid, accessed 11th December 2018.
- Boyles, Salynn, 'Folic Acid in Utero Tied to Food Allergy Risk', *Medpage Today* (March 2018), https://www.medpagetoday.com/meetingcoverage/aaaai/71566, accessed 11th December 2018.
- British Dietetic Association, 'Food Fact Sheet: Folic Acid' (August 2016), https://www.bda.uk.com/foodfacts/FolicAcid.pdf, accessed 11th December 2018.
- Business Wire, 'Prota/MCRI Completes Enrolment of Phase 2b Multicentre Clinical Trial of Probiotic Oral Immunotherapy for the Treatment of Peanut Allergy (PPOIT-003)' (May 2018), https://www.businesswire.com/news/home/20180522006495/en/ProtaMCRI-Completes-Enrolment-Phase-2b-Multicentre-Clinical
- Fox, A and Meyer, R, 'How close are we to revolutionising the prevention and dietary management of food allergy?' *Nutrica Expert Opinion Webinar* (May 2018), https://www.nutriciacongresses.com/congresses/presentation/148/how-close-are-we-to-revolutionising-the-prevention-and-dietary-management-of-food-allergy--/, accessed 9th October 2018.
- Kresser, Chris, 'The little known (but crucial) difference between folate and folic acid' (March 2012), https://chriskresser.com/folate-vs-folic-acid/
- Leech, Joe, 'L-Methylfolate (5-MTHF): Your Must-Read Beginner's Guide', *Diet vs. disease* (May 2018), https://www.dietvsdisease.org/l-methylfolate-5-mthf/, accessed 11th December 2018.
- Medical Xpress, 'Food allergy is linked to skin exposure and genetics' (April 2018), https://medicalxpress.com/news/2018-04-food-allergy-

linked-skin-exposure.html, accessed 11ᵗʰ December 2018.

- National Institutes of Health, 'Skin patch to treat peanut allergy shows benefit in children' (October 2016), https://www.nih.gov/news-events/news-releases/skin-patch-treat-peanut-allergy-shows-benefit-children, accessed 11ᵗʰ December 2018.

- New Scientist, 'Probiotics and fish oil in pregnancy may reduce child allergies' (February 2018), https://www.newscientist.com/article/2162590-probiotics-and-fish-oil-in-pregnancy-may-reduce-child-allergies/, accessed 11ᵗʰ December 2018.

- NHS, 'Probiotics and fish oil in pregnancy may reduce allergies in children' (March 2018), https://www.nhs.uk/news/pregnancy-and-child/probiotics-and-fish-oil-in-pregnancy-may-reduce-allergies-children/, accessed 11ᵗʰ December 2018.

- OITCenter.com, 'What is Oral Immunotherapy?' (2012), http://www.oitcenter.com/oit.htm, accessed 11ᵗʰ December 2018.

- Papadopoulos, Nikos, 'When and how should oral immunotherapy for food allergy become daily clinical practice?' [slideshow] (November 2017), https://www.anaphylaxis.org.uk/wp-content/uploads/2017/11/When-and-how-should-oral-immunotherapy-for-food-allergy-become-daily-clinical-practice-by-Nikolaos-G.-Papadopoulos.pdf, accessed 11ᵗʰ December 2018.

- Nørhede, Pia, 'Food allergy diagnosis today and in the future' *European Academy of Allergy and Clinical Immunology* (n.d.), http://www.eaaci.org/food-allergy/Food-allergy-diagnosis-today-and-in-the-future.pdf, accessed 11ᵗʰ December 2018.

CHAPTER 12

THE TEENAGE YEARS

The teenage years are an exciting time with many new experiences for your child. Your teen will go through many transitions as they gradually progress to adulthood. This is a period of massive brain development, alongside puberty with its hormones and physical changes.

This process can cause unpredictable behaviour and emotions, which can be demanding for parents and children to deal with. At the same time, as teenagers become more independent from their parents, their peer relationships become more important to them. Being a teenager with food allergies adds an additional challenge along the way.

If a child hasn't outgrown their food allergies by the beginning of the teenage years, they will most likely have them for life. For parents this means it is important to keep educating your teenager about their food allergies and increasingly encourage them to take over day-to-day management themselves.

BRAIN DEVELOPMENT AND BEHAVIOUR

Children's brains undergo a lot of growth and change as they become teenagers. This continues until the mid-twenties, and will affect your child's thinking and behaviour. The prefrontal cortex is the part of the brain associated with planning, understanding the consequences of actions, problem solving and impulse control, and is the last part of the brain to become fully developed. While it is still developing, teenagers rely more on a different part of the brain called the amygdala, which is more instinctual and less logical, for making decisions and solving problems. As your child develops, you may notice that sometimes they seem quite mature but at other times they may still be impulsive, illogical or emotional.

Adolescents are also very egocentric and often seem to believe the world revolves around them. They think a lot about how other people see them and they may change their behaviour depending on how they think their friends will perceive it. Peer relationships become very important to them, and parental influence decreases. They may feel very self-conscious in social situations. Teenagers often believe that they, and their feelings, are special and unique. They may even believe they are invincible. As they get older they will begin to realise that other people may not be as interested in them as they are themselves!

During this time, it is normal to see your child taking more risks than usual, experimenting with new things, being more emotional, and making impulsive decisions. This is all a healthy part of them creating their own independent identity, but it also means they need to be aware of how to keep themselves safe without relying on you. In addition, your child will gradually become more able to think abstractly, empathise with others, plan ahead and solve problems.

TEACHING YOUR TEEN ABOUT FOOD ALLERGIES

If your child was diagnosed with food allergies at a young age they will be used to not being allowed to eat certain foods, having to bring their own food with them and taking extra precautions such as washing hands before and after eating. To be able to manage their own food allergies independently, they will need more information about food allergies, in a way that they can understand. This will mean many small conversations over the years, rather than one big talk.

They need to know about their individual level of risk. Explain the symptoms they may experience if they have an allergic reaction, as well as the precautions they need to take to keep themselves safe. Think about your teen's personality and level of understanding as you discuss this – but make sure these are established as non-negotiable boundaries. Find the right balance between giving them the knowledge they need to take their allergies seriously, without making them overly anxious. You can help by providing a role model of being careful but not fearful.

At the same time, your teen can take on a more active role in managing their own allergies. You will need to accept that you are no longer in control of every situation, and that your child may want to find their own way of doing things. You will need to give them many opportunities to practise, so get them involved when shopping for food and eating out, show them how to read labels and allergen menus, and encourage them to order food themselves. You can start by trying things out at home, role playing different situations that may arise, allowing them to rehearse expressing their needs, and take baby steps towards doing things in the real world. They will need to practise assertiveness in a variety of circumstances, such as being able to politely turn down unsafe foods, saying no to unsafe situations and being specific about what they need.

In order to advocate for themselves, they will need to be aware of exactly which foods are unsafe for them and what they look like, both at the supermarket and when eating out. They will need to be able to ask questions about food given to them to make sure it is safe, and how to ask for help if they start to feel unwell. If they have an epinephrine auto-injector they will need to know to always carry it, when to use it, how to administer it themselves, and how to call an ambulance. Teach them to always err on the side of caution – so if they think they may be having a reaction, to take their medicine and ask for medical help, even if they are not completely sure. Ideally, start teaching them all this while they are still at primary school so it is well established.

As well as teaching them the skills and knowledge they need, make sure your teen has plenty of opportunities to talk about any problems they are having. They will need to talk about practical issues but also give them time to express how they feel about their allergies. Having to be constantly vigilant is a big emotional burden for a young person to deal with. Having food allergies may be the biggest challenge they have ever had to deal with in their lives so far, and at times it can be stressful. It may also make them feel different and isolated from their peers – but you can explain that everyone feels different in some way. Life would be very boring if we were all the same! The good news is that learning to overcome these difficulties in adolescence will make them more resilient and empathetic towards others as adults. See also Chapter 15 for more ideas about stress management for both you and your child.

Teenagers may not always volunteer information, so it's up to you to keep the lines of communication open. Ask open-ended questions about their day such as who they are hanging out with and what they have been up to. This can help to give you a sense of how well they are managing their allergies, how friendships are developing, and if romantic relationships are starting.

When your teenager does come up against practical problems, or when they encounter a new situation, see it as an opportunity for you to teach them problem solving strategies. Be wary of simply telling them what to do, as this doesn't encourage them to think for themselves (and there's no guarantee that they will do what you suggest anyway!). Instead, see if you can encourage your teen to come up with solutions themselves, perhaps brainstorming potential ideas with them and allowing them to make the final decision about how they will handle it. Acknowledge when your child acts responsibly and makes good decisions about handling their food allergies. Sometimes mistakes will happen. This is a normal part of the learning process and is not anybody's fault. It is important to talk about what went wrong and what to do differently in future to prevent the same thing happening again. Make sure you deal with your own feelings before speaking to your child so that you can remain calm.

With a positive attitude and some extra forethought, if there is something your teenager really wants to do, they never have to let food allergies stop them. You want your child to have as many opportunities and experiences in life as possible, and so you have to find a way to make it safe. Listen to your child. They will let you know what is important to them. Sometimes they may act like they don't care but this can be because they feel overwhelmed.

Teenagers love to be spontaneous and you will need to come up with strategies to manage this together. For example, it is useful for them to have good knowledge of which restaurants in their local area are safe for them to eat at, as well as how to explain to their friends why it is important to eat there. You can go online together to check allergen menus and make a list of safe restaurants, or download a mobile app such as Biteappy or Libereat to check restaurants on-the-go. You can show them how to patch test foods against their own skin (if it is safe to do so). You can also encourage them to always have safe snacks with them in case of an unexpected situation.

Teach your teenager how to cook. This is an important life skill for anyone to learn, but especially so for those with food allergies who are unable to rely on convenience foods or takeaways. If they can learn to feed themselves safely, their independence will increase. You can also practise shopping for food and reading food labels, and it is good to start this early, with you still there to provide help and guidance. Apps like FoodMaestro and Libereat have barcode scanners, which can be an additional check when they are getting started with this.

Sometimes teenagers will be more receptive to information if it comes from a source other than their parents. You could ask another family member or friend to speak to your child. Or it could be their dietitian or doctor. You may want to give them time during an appointment to talk to a health professional without you there. Another source of information could be from the internet. There are some great resources about allergies specifically for teens such as:

- Anaphylaxis UK: Young People
  https://www.anaphylaxis.org.uk/young-people/
- Why Risk It (Canadian website) http://www.whyriskit.ca/ and smartphone app

- Ultimate Guidebook for Teens with Allergies (Canadian) http://www.whyriskit.ca/ultimate-guidebook.html
- Food Allergy Research & Education: Resources for Teens (American website) https://www.foodallergy.org/education-awareness/community-resources/resources-for-teens
- YouTube can also be a good source of information but remember to watch videos yourself before showing them to your teen to check they are suitable
- Social media – look for official allergy charities such as Allergy UK and Anaphylaxis UK

SECONDARY SCHOOL

When your child transitions to secondary school you will need to put in place an allergy management plan as described in Chapter 8. Secondary school is very different to primary school, with a larger building, more pupils, less adult supervision at breaktimes and lunchtimes, and different teachers for each subject. There is also a wider range of after-school activities which may go on into the evening, as well as school trips and possible travel abroad.

Because your child will be moving around the school for different lessons, you will need to consider issues such as where emergency medication such as epinephrine auto-injectors or asthma inhalers will be stored or carried. All of your child's teachers should know where the emergency medication is, and they may wish to carry out 'spot-checks' to ensure that your child is carrying their medication. Schools may be able to keep spares in the school office and in the canteen if necessary. Ideally, all school staff should be informed about all allergic students and receive allergy training, including teachers and kitchen staff, because a reaction could happen outside of lesson time.

Moving on to secondary school also means your teenager will lose touch with some of their old friends who knew them well and knew about their allergies, and start making new friends. Children at this age may be reluctant to tell their new friends about their allergies because they just want to fit in and they don't want to be seen as different. Discuss with your child who needs to know about their allergies, how to bring up the subject, and what they should tell people.

You will need to make sure the school has safe seating arrangements at lunchtimes, such as a nut-free table, or making sure your child has a designated table to sit at which will be wiped down by kitchen staff before they eat. Your child will need to check ingredients at the school canteen every time they buy food. They may be more comfortable bringing a packed lunch, so they know the food is safe and so that they don't have to draw attention to themselves by asking questions of canteen staff.

You can also ask for the school to include a special lesson to raise awareness of food allergies within the school community. This does not have to mention your child specifically, but would give other children important information that can help to keep your child safe, such as what is a food allergy, how to spot an allergic reaction and what to do in an emergency. It can also encourage empathy in others by making them aware of how much care and attention it takes to prevent a reaction, which can help to reduce allergy bullying (see later in this chapter for more on dealing with bullying).

For school trips, work with the school to create a risk assessment and plan of action. Ask the teacher organising the trip for a detailed itinerary. For overnight trips, call ahead to hotels and restaurants to inform them of your child's allergies and make arrangements for meals. Pack plenty of safe snacks and extra money for your teen in case of delay or emergency. Go through the itinerary with your child and think of any potential pitfalls and how to deal with them. For your own peace of mind, you can ask your child to text home after every meal, even if just to say 'ok'. Give all the teachers going on the trip written information about:

- Medication needs
- Itinerary and meal arrangements, including managers' names
- How much help your child needs with things like reading food labels and ordering food (a 17-year-old will be more independent than a 13-year-old, for example)

- Any parts of the trip they will need to skip or avoid
- Your mobile phone number in case of any questions

SOCIAL LIFE

As a child moves into the teenage years, old friendships may fade away and new ones are formed. Friendships become more stable at this age, with teenagers often falling into regular groups of friends that they prefer to spend time with.

A teenager's social life has much less adult supervision than a younger child. Teenagers with food allergies will need to learn how to be vigilant for themselves. They will need to be assertive and able to resist peer pressure.

You could help your child to make a checklist for leaving the house and display it near the front door or in their bedroom, or keep it in their bag. For example, epinephrine, inhalers, baby wipes (for hands), snacks, money, phone. Or alternatively, make up an allergy kit in a smaller bag or pencil case that can be grabbed on the way out the door, or slipped into a larger bag.

As your child makes new friends, at some point they will need to talk to them about their allergies. Role playing can be really helpful to prepare for this so your child can develop a short 'speech' that they can give whenever the topic arises with new people. Let your child decide which friends need to know such as their best friends, people they eat lunch with and so on. They can let this come up naturally, it doesn't need to be a big deal. Remember, many people have a special situation that needs empathy from their friends. Alternatively, your teenager can use social media or text messages to share information about allergies with their friends, such as videos or photos of allergic reactions.

If you and your child both want to, you could host an 'Epi-Pen party', where your child invites their friends over to socialise, and you can spend a short time teaching them about allergies, perhaps using an age-appropriate video, and show them how to use an auto-injector. Many children with food allergies find it empowering to teach others and raise awareness of their condition.

When your child is visiting their friends' houses without you, you will need to speak to the parents about your child's allergies. Some parents will be willing and able to manage your child's allergies, others may not. Sometimes it might be safer to host gatherings and sleepovers yourself.

ALCOHOL

In the UK, the average age that teenagers try alcohol for the first time is now 13.3 years, and drinking is seen as a normal part of teenage life and growing up, especially for older teenagers. It's important for all teenagers to learn how to drink responsibly but there are additional risks for those with food allergies. Some drinks contain allergens – for example cream-based liqueurs contain dairy, and beer contains gluten, so it's important to be aware of what you are drinking. Alcoholic drinks do not have to be labelled with food allergens, which can make it very tricky.

For parties it may be safer to take their own drinks – this also helps to limit how much they drink. Don't share drinks with other people as there is a risk of cross-contact – this includes drinking games. In addition, if teenagers are drinking, they may be less careful about checking what they are eating, and become unable to keep themselves safe. Make them aware that epinephrine is less effective if you have been drinking. Your teen may even decide they prefer not to drink because of the risk of losing control.

DATING

At some point your child will start dating and they will need to speak to their dates about their food allergy. This might come up naturally if your teenager wants to go to a restaurant on a date. Or they may need to pick a time to speak to their potential date about it. It's better to do it sooner rather than later, and get it out of the way. Again, it can be helpful to practise in advance what they want to say.

Teenagers also need to know that if they kiss someone who has recently (within a few hours) eaten the food they are allergic to, it could cause a reaction. They will need to discuss this with their partner. It is difficult to bring up in the heat of the moment, so although it might feel awkward, it's important to mention it early on in a relationship. If they haven't talked about it, then no kissing. To prevent kiss reactions, waiting at least 5 hours after eating the allergen can help, along with eating another meal in between, and brushing teeth.

Hopefully most people will react positively to this information and if they care about your teenager they will be willing to make adjustments. It's possible to have fun dates without food. If boyfriends or girlfriends are unsympathetic or careless, unfortunately this means it is time to move on. Your teenager's health and safety are more important than any relationship. This can actually be a good way of weeding out unsuitable partners early on! Explain to your teen that, if someone really wants to be with them, they won't want to do anything that could make them feel unwell.

BULLYING

Food allergy bullying happens to about a third of teenagers with food allergies, so it's an issue that parents need to be aware of. It can be dangerous and must be taken seriously, as other teens may tease or threaten your child with foods they are allergic to.

Teenagers may not always tell you when they are being bullied. This is where maintaining regular communication using open-ended questions and listening carefully to responses is really helpful. You may get a hint that someone is picking on them, or if they refuse to talk to you, that can be another sign of a problem. If they open up to you that they are being bullied, give them a chance to talk about how it has made them feel.

Work with your teen to make an action plan to address the bullying. Is there a friend they could talk to, or a teacher they trust? Can they avoid the bully? How will they respond to the bully?

At the same time, try to strengthen existing friendships by inviting children round after school or organising other social gatherings.

Encourage them to take part in activities outside of school so that they can make friends outside their normal circle.

If the bullying is happening at school, contact the school and make them aware of what has happened, including specific times and places. They may be able to increase supervision so that the bully gets caught in the act, and it is not just your child's word against theirs. You can also ask for the bully to be moved to a different table or class. Keep a diary of any incidents your child reports. If you feel that the school are not doing enough, you can write to the headteacher to complain. If the bully has caused your child to have an allergic reaction, contact the police as this is assault and is a criminal offence.

It is also important to be aware of cyber bullying. Social networking sites all have policies against bullying behaviours. If it happens, take a screenshot of the comment or photo and send it to the site, along with the terms and conditions that have been breached. You can also block or unfollow the person on the site, or increase privacy settings to prevent people seeing information you don't want them to see, and stop unwanted messages. For text messages, you can block the phone number of anyone who is bothering you. Don't reply to any nasty messages or comments online – sometimes a reaction is what the bully wants.

The teenage years bring new challenges for all children to contend with. Teenagers with food allergies must also learn how to manage their condition themselves. It can be difficult for parents to handle too, as it can feel strange to let go of control. Make time to fully prepare your teen for dealing with different situations that they may encounter in life, so they are ready to move into adulthood.

KEY POINTS

- Children undergo a huge amount of developmental changes during the teenage years. This can affect their moods and behaviour and they may seem unpredictable.
- Teach your teen everything they need to know about managing their own food allergies. This is a gradual process which happens in small steps.

- Communicate with their secondary school and put an allergy management plan in place.
- Encourage your teen to develop their own strategies for managing their social life.
- Watch out for signs of bullying and take action if it does happen to your child.

REFERENCES

- Raising Children, 'Brain development: teenagers' (December 2017), http://raisingchildren.net.au/articles/brain_development_teenagers.html, accessed 11th December 2018.
- Elkind, David, 'Egocentrism in Adolesence', *Child Development*, 38, 4 (1967), doi: 10.2307/1127100.
- Hewett, Heather, 'Food Allergy Meets the Teenage Brain', *Allergic Living* (November 2015), https://www.allergicliving.com/2015/11/23/food-allergy-meets-the-teenage-brain/, accessed 11th December 2018.
- Drink Aware, 'Teenage drinking' (n.d.), https://www.drinkaware.co.uk/advice/underage-drinking/teenage-drinking/, accessed 11th December 2018.

CHAPTER 13

UNIVERSITY

If your child has the opportunity to go to university, take it! Don't allow food allergies to hold them back. Admittedly, it is a new challenge as your son or daughter will be going to a new place, possibly hundreds of miles from home, where they don't know anyone and no one knows about their food allergies. However, it is such a fantastic experience and food allergies should never stop your child from doing anything they want to do. Although it can be hard to let go, at the age of eighteen, your child will be an adult capable of looking after themselves.

You and your child will need to do lots of careful planning and preparation together before they leave for university. But remember that everyone has a difficulty to overcome. Some people may be struggling to get the exam results they need. Others may have financial worries. Some people may have learning difficulties or a mobility issue. Keep a positive attitude and don't be disheartened.

MAKING A SHORTLIST

Encourage your child to research universities based on what they want from the experience first and foremost. There are over 150 universities in the UK and each one is different. What subject they want to study should be the first consideration, but you will also need to think about whether they want a campus or city university, and other things like sports provision, work placements, travel abroad, flexible courses and so on. It's a good idea to visit a few universities to get a feel for each one as they are all very different.

Then, think about what additional requirements your child will need in order to accommodate their food allergy. Not every university will be able to deliver everything you need – it depends what facilities they have available. Some universities are more clued up than others and may already have an allergy policy or staff with allergy training. However, if you can't get the right provisions for your child's needs, it may rule out some options. Read this chapter together with your son or daughter and work out exactly what their needs are.

CATERING

There is a lot of variation in catering provision between universities. Most universities have a traditional cafeteria but many will also have additional food outlets including coffee shops, sandwich bars, takeaways, cafes, bars and restaurants. Can you find somewhere on site that can cater for you? Visiting the campus on an open day can really help you to see what different universities can offer.

University cafeterias and restaurants are subject to the same food allergen laws as all restaurants, so they have to provide you with information on food allergens when you ask for it (see Chapter 6 for more detail).

Speak to the catering staff to find out if they can cater for you. You might be the first person going to that university with severe allergies so be prepared to educate them. Tell them every possible food you could be allergic to – for example don't just say 'dairy' but explain that this includes milk, cheese, cream, ice cream, butter and so on. Be honest and detailed about what you need as you will be relying on them to cook for you during your time at university. If they are not able to meet your needs you will need to look into alternative solutions, like self-catering accommodation.

In addition to the usual self-service cafeteria, possible options that the university may be able to provide include:

- Pre-ordered meals, where you choose in advance from a menu of options and the food is ready for you when you arrive.
- Allergy-friendly stations, where all the food on a particular station is allergen-free.
- Short-order stations, where they will prepare your food to order.
- Allergy-friendly pre-prepared food, where food is always available – this can be a good option for cold food like sandwiches.

If the cafeteria is not able to cater for you, find out if they will allow you to bring your own food to eat there, so that you can still sit with your friends.

ACCOMMODATION

For a person with food allergies, having access to a kitchen is a non-negotiable requirement. Think about the minimum you will need such as a fridge and microwave. Can the university provide this in halls of residence or will you need to seek private accommodation? Arrange your accommodation early to ensure you get something suitable.

When choosing accommodation, consider who else will be using the kitchen. Students are often messy and a house share with strangers is risky – at the very least it may mean cleaning up after other people before you can start preparing your own food. Sharing a house might be easier to manage in the second and third years of your course where you can live with people you already know. Maybe you would prefer to share with only one or two friends, to reduce the risk. When you are choosing housemates, be upfront about your allergies. If they are not willing to make adaptations for you, don't live with them – it's not worth the risk.

You may feel it is safer to live in a single or studio apartment, especially if you have multiple or very severe allergies. You can control allergens much better if you are the only person using the kitchen. It doesn't have to be isolating, as you could just use your apartment as a base for sleeping and preparing food – you don't have to spend all your time there! The downside is that if you were to have a reaction at home, you would be alone.

LOCATION

As well as the campus itself, you will need to consider the general location of the university. Are there restaurants you can eat at safely in the town or city of your university? Is there a GP surgery on campus? A pharmacy where you can collect prescriptions? Is there a hospital nearby? How long would it take an ambulance to get to campus? What supermarkets are nearby and are they accessible by public transport?

APPLYING TO UNIVERSITY

You can declare any disabilities, including food allergies, on your UCAS form. This is partly so that UCAS can collect statistics on different student groups, but also so that universities can help you if you need it. When you start to get offers, the disability departments at the university may use this information to get in touch with you and find out what you need. You don't have to tell them, but if the university doesn't know about your allergy, they can't take steps to keep you safe. It will not have any bearing on your academic application. You are protected against discrimination by law.

Under the Equality Act 2010, a disability is defined as "a physical or mental impairment" that "has a substantial and long-term adverse effect on a person's ability to do normal day-to-day activities". If you have been admitted to hospital in the past for anaphylactic shock, your allergies are potentially life threatening, and you have had to adapt your life to accommodate your allergies, then this would likely be classed as a disability. This means that it is against the law for universities to discriminate against you, such as excluding you from a course or a course trip because of your food allergies. Universities also have to make 'reasonable adjustments' so that you are not put at a disadvantage.

INFORMING THE UNIVERSITY

Once you have accepted an offer, you must talk to your university's disability support department about your food allergies well before you start your course so that they have time to put any arrangements in place. You may need to request that your course tutors have allergy training so that they know what to do in an emergency. You might also need to ask that other students on your course do not eat your allergen immediately before your lectures or seminars. They may need to make changes to your accommodation, such as deep-cleaning it over the summer holidays before you arrive, replacing furniture or kitchen equipment, or providing you with a mini-fridge or microwave.

Make sure the manager or chef at the cafeteria you want to use is made aware of your allergies so that they can plan ahead. They may need time to make adjustments for you such as training their staff. The university may be able to liaise with catering staff for you, or you may prefer to meet with them personally.

FINANCES

Being on a special diet will increase your food costs, compared to other students. You will need to learn how to manage your budget, plan meals, and shop frugally. If necessary, get a part time job to earn extra income. You are very unlikely to get additional financial support for food allergies. The Disabled Students Allowances cover additional costs incurred as a direct result of a disability, learning difficulty or health condition – but only costs that are directly related to studying. Some universities provide additional funding that you may be able to access if you are struggling financially, such as hardship funds. You will need to speak to the individual university to find out what they can offer.

PREPARING YOUR TEENAGER FOR UNIVERSITY LIFE

Students are at a high risk when they first arrive at university because they want to fit in and may not want to ask questions about what is in their food, so you must reinforce the importance of carrying medication and being assertive to your son or daughter before they leave. Give them lots of opportunities to practice when out and about in the months before they go to university, if they are not already.

You will also need to ensure your student can shop and cook for themselves. This includes knowing how to read food labels and being able to store and prepare food safely in a shared kitchen. They will need to be aware of how much time they need to allow to do this, especially if they will be reliant on public transport. You could make a personalised recipe book for them to take with them, teaching them how to cook all the meals before they leave. Giving them lots of practice means they can prove to themselves that they are ready to manage their allergies on their own, and advocate for themselves.

Practice explaining food allergies so that they are comfortable telling people about it. Help them prepare a short spiel that they can use when meeting new people if that helps. Discuss potential situations that could arise and how to deal with them, for example if friends want to eat at an unsafe restaurant, would you try and persuade them to go somewhere else, ask the restaurant if you can bring your own food, or meet your friends after the meal for a drink?

STAYING SAFE AT UNIVERSITY

Once your child is at university they are considered an adult, so they will be responsible for carrying their own medication. Have a medicine bag such as a clear pencil case which contains all their emergency medication along with their emergency plan, which can be slipped inside or clipped onto a larger bag. If possible, have several of these and keep them in different locations e.g. keep one in their back pack, one in their room, one in their gym bag etc. This makes it harder to accidentally forget their medicine, and if one gets lost they still have others as back up. Make sure they practise using their auto-injector so that they will be able to use it if a reaction happens.

Before they leave, encourage them to talk to their doctor about their emergency plan so that they become in charge of it. You will need to give them responsibility for it, and they will need to make sure they are familiar with it and keep it up to date. They may like to download a mobile phone app such as AllergyMe which can be used to alert others in an emergency situation.

In shared accommodation, your child will need to tell all their housemates about their food allergy, what to do in case of an emergency, where they keep your medication, and what they need to do to keep them safe. It can be helpful for each individual to have their own cupboard and fridge shelf to keep food separate. High shelves are better to avoid cross-contact. Your child could also use sticky labels to mark their safe foods, or if they're really worried, keep non-perishable food in their room. Ongoing communication is really important too. People do make mistakes and when this happens your child must tell them immediately – it's easy for people to forget when it's not their own issue.

Your child will also have to plan ahead for social events where food will be served. They can either speak to the organiser to make arrangements, eat beforehand, or bring their own food. They should always ask questions and never eat food if they're not sure it's safe.

Once you and your child have made all the necessary arrangements to accommodate their food allergy, they should be able to make the most of university life without having to worry too much. It will probably be harder for you as than it is for them as they become fully independent and start living away from home, managing their allergy themselves. Once they settle in it will become a normal part of their daily routine and lifestyle.

KEY POINTS

- Look at what catering options different universities can provide.
- Think about what accommodation will suit your needs.
- Decide whether the general location of the university is suitable.
- Tell the university about your food allergy – both the disability department and the catering team.

- Plan how to meet the extra financial costs of living with food allergies on a student budget.
- Prepare for shopping and cooking independently.
- Practice talking to people about food allergies and asking questions.
- Be ready to let your child take charge of managing their food allergies for themselves.

REFERENCES AND LINKS

- Bunning, Denise A., 'From Sleepovers to College: Coaching Your Food Allergic Child to Independence' [video], *Food Allergy Research & Education* (May 2017) https://www.youtube.com/watch?v=b9CZjP9nWu0, accessed 13th July 2018.
- Gov.uk, 'Equality Act 2010: guidance' (June 2015), https://www.gov.uk/guidance/equality-act-2010-guidance
- Grim, Kristi, 'Dorm Life and Dining Plans: Planning for College with Food Allergies' [video], *Food Allergy Research & Education'* (April 2015), https://www.youtube.com/watch?v=2dm1yXGYMBQ
- Roth, Lily, 'Navigating College and the college process with food allergies' [video], *Food Allergy Research & Education* (July 2017), https://www.youtube.com/watch?v=ZeFXkuMDnDQ
- Stevenson, Charlotte, 'The scariest thing about leaving home? My severe nut allergy', *The Guardian* (July 2017), https://www.theguardian.com/education/2017/jul/07/how-to-cope-with-severe-allergies-nuts-university, accessed 3rd June 2018
- The Complete University Guide, 'Choosing a University' (n.d.), https://www.thecompleteuniversityguide.co.uk/universities/choosing-the-right-university/
- UCAS, 'Disabled Students' (n.d.), https://www.ucas.com/undergraduate/applying-university/individual-needs/disabled-students

CHAPTER 14

FOOD ALLERGY MYTH BUSTING

Awareness of food allergies is growing, but many people still hold some misconceptions. It can be hard to understand what it is like to live with food allergies if you have never experienced it yourself. Here are some common myths around food allergies.

MYTH: A food intolerance is the same as a food allergy, just less severe.

FALSE: A food allergy is when the body's immune system reacts to a food that is normally harmless. An intolerance is caused by an inability to digest the food in question and does not involve the immune system. Allergic reactions can range from mild (e.g. diarrhoea) to potentially life threatening. People with allergies may have a reaction to even a tiny amount of the food they are allergic to, whereas people with an intolerance may still be able to eat the food in small quantities.

MYTH: If you think you have a food allergy or intolerance, you should cut the food out of your diet straight away.

FALSE: You should speak to your GP first. There are other conditions that can have similar symptoms to food allergies. You may need to have tests to diagnose the problem or rule out other conditions. For example, coeliac disease causes unpleasant symptoms after eating foods containing gluten. It can be diagnosed by a blood test but only while you are still eating gluten regularly.

MYTH: Food allergies are becoming more common.

TRUE: The number of children admitted to hospital for food-related anaphylaxis has increased by 700% since 1990. 1 in 13 children now have a food allergy. This is roughly 2 children in every school classroom. This number is expected to increase even more into the future.

MYTH: You can only be allergic to certain foods.

FALSE: You can be allergic to any food. However, some food allergies are more common than others. In the UK, these common allergens cause 90% of allergic reactions. These are: celery, cereals containing gluten (e.g. wheat, rye, barley and oats), crustaceans (e.g. crabs and prawns), eggs, fish, lupin, milk, molluscs (e.g. mussels and oysters), mustard, tree nuts, peanuts, sesame seeds, soya, sulphur dioxide or sulphites.

MYTH: Allergic reactions always happen immediately after eating the food.

FALSE: Symptoms of an allergic reaction may happen immediately or can be delayed and only appear several hours later. See chapter 1 for more details on immediate and delayed reactions.

MYTH: Food allergies are not a serious problem.

FALSE: A severe allergic reaction (anaphylaxis) can kill if it isn't treated immediately. So people with severe allergies must always carry their medication with them wherever they go. In the UK, about ten people die every year from food-induced anaphylaxis. Food allergies also have a huge impact on a person's quality of life, as well as the rest of their family, because they must always be careful to avoid a reaction. This is a continuous burden which affects every aspect of daily life.

MYTH: Most children grow out of their allergies.

MAYBE: Just over a quarter of children grow out of their allergies. Children have a good chance of outgrowing allergies to egg, milk, wheat and soya. However, allergies to peanuts, seafood, fish and tree nuts are usually lifelong.

MYTH: If you have a food allergy you can only have a reaction by eating the food.

FALSE: Some people will react on skin contact with the allergen, or react to particles of dust in the air. Some cosmetics may contain food allergens and could cause a reaction if they come into contact with the body. For example, soaps and shampoos sometimes contain almond oil or milk. The injectable flu vaccine is not suitable for people with severe egg allergy. Some medicines are made with peanut oil.

MYTH: A little bit won't hurt.

FALSE: Some children can have an allergic reaction to even a tiny amount of food. Even a tiny crumb could be enough to cause an allergic reaction in some children. If your child has a food allergy you should strictly avoid the food, until advised to reintroduce it by a medical professional.

MYTH: You can self-diagnose a food allergy.

FALSE: Around 30% of people believe they are allergic or intolerant to one or more foods, but it is estimated that only 5-8% of children and 1-2% of adults have a clinical food allergy. Always speak to your GP if you think your child has a food allergy, before taking any foods out of their diet.

MYTH: You can diagnose food allergy with a home test kit.

FALSE: Food allergies can only be diagnosed by speaking to a medical professional, who may recommend tests such as a blood test or skin prick test (see Chapter 2). They will explain how to interpret your results with consideration of your symptoms and medical history. Home tests such as vega tests, applied kinesiology, hair analysis and IgG blood tests do not give reliable results.

MYTH: Food additives and artificial flavours are the most common causes of food allergic reactions.

FALSE: It is possible, but rare, to be allergic to food additives and artificial flavours. Natural foods cause most allergic reactions.

MYTH: Anyone can develop a food allergy.

TRUE: But you are more likely to develop a food allergy if you have eczema or asthma, or if someone else in your immediate family has eczema, asthma or any type of allergy.

MYTH: Each allergic reaction will be worse than the last one.

FALSE: Allergic reactions can be different every time. There's no way to know if a reaction will be mild, moderate or severe. It's impossible to predict how your body will react. This is why it's important to keep your emergency medication with you all the time (if prescribed), just in case.

MYTH: Peanut is the most common food allergy in children.

FALSE: Milk is the most common food allergy in children, followed by eggs.

MYTH: Peanuts are the 'worst' food allergy.

FALSE: Any food can cause an allergy, and any allergy can cause a severe reaction. Every individual is different. However, peanut allergy is the most likely to result in severe, possible life-threatening reactions.

MYTH: Food allergies always develop in childhood.

FALSE: Food allergies are more common in children than adults, but you can develop a food allergy at any age, even to a food you've eaten safely before.

MYTH: Food allergies or intolerances can be cured.

FALSE: The only way to prevent a reaction is to avoid the food you are allergic to. Research is being done into treatments for food allergies but these are still at an early stage. Children sometimes grow out of their allergies naturally as they develop and their immune systems mature.

REFERENCES AND LINKS

- Food Standards Agency, 'Food allergy facts' (n.d.), http://allergytraining.food.gov.uk/english/food-allergy-facts.aspx, accessed 11th December 2018.
- Food Allergy Research & Education, 'Food Allergy Myths And Misconceptions' (n.d.), https://www.foodallergy.org/life-with-food-allergies/food-allergy-101/food-allergy-myths-and-misconceptions, accessed 11th December 2018.
- Stöppler, Melissa Conrad, '5 Food Allergy Myths', *MedicineNet* (July 2017), https://www.medicinenet.com/5_food_allergy_myths/views.htm, accessed 11th December 2018.
- NHS Choices, 'Food allergy and intolerance myth buster' (2014) https://www.nhs.uk/Tools/Documents/Food%20allergy%20and%20intolerance%20myth%20buster.htm, accessed 17th February 2018.

CHAPTER 15

EMOTIONS

Managing food allergies places extra demands on parents. You have to be vigilant all the time when you have a child with food allergies, and normal day-to-day activities need extra preparedness. Feeling excluded causes social stress. Many people misunderstand food allergies and do not take them seriously. The fear of having a reaction may be always in the back of your mind. Having severe or multiple food allergies has been shown to have a similar effect on quality of life as other long-term health conditions such as Type I diabetes or epilepsy. In additional to the practical aspects of managing food allergy, you must take into consideration the emotional impact on the whole family.

YOUR EMOTIONS

Having a child with food allergies is a journey and you may experience different emotional reactions along the way. The beginning is the most difficult time, when everything is new. As you learn about food allergies and change your habits things gradually become easier over time. However, certain events in life can trigger more stress along the way.

If you are waiting for diagnosis, you may feel a lot of uncertainty. It can take time as you wait for referrals, appointments and test results. You may be unsure of what is wrong with your child, what is causing their symptoms, and wondering if it will ever get better. Health professionals aren't always clued up about allergies which can make things even more stressful and long-winded. If your child has had a severe reaction, it can be really scary for you to witness. Allow time to process your emotions and talk to others about how you are feeling.

When your child is newly diagnosed, learning about and managing their allergies will take up a lot of your time and attention. There is an adjustment period. You will have a lot of information to absorb all at once and have to change family eating habits. Family members may not all agree on the best way to do this!

Try not to make your family life revolve around your child's allergies. Remember to have fun and do things that you all enjoy. Try activities that don't revolve around food such as a visit to the beach, going for a walk in the woods or a trip to a museum. Gradually start to try situations that you are worried about such as attending a children's birthday party or going out for a meal in a restaurant, to build up confidence.

You may feel sad that your child cannot eat certain foods that you enjoy and that you will miss out on that shared experience. For example, it might not be possible to take your child out for ice cream. You may need time to process a sense of loss. But remember that food is not the most important thing in life and there are many, many ways to have fun without food being the main focus.

Remember to take good care of yourself. Make time to do things that make you feel happy, that do not revolve around your child or their allergies. We all know the importance of self-care. It might sound back-to-front, but as a busy parent with children relying on you, looking after yourself is even more important. You are not just a parent of a child with food allergies but also a spouse, employee, sibling, friend, volunteer... Burning out is not an option!

Keep a positive attitude. For all intents and purposes, your child is a healthy, normal child who will grow and develop in the same way as their peers. It's not always easy but if your child wants to do something, you can find a way for them to do it. Think of positive aspects of food allergies. For example, you will probably eat much more healthily if you are unable to rely on packaged food. Your cooking skills will improve. When relatives and friends make the effort to learn about allergies and keep your child safe, it can actually strengthen relationships.

You may also feel guilty at times. You may worry that you did something to cause your child's allergies. You may feel responsible if you have accidentally given your child a food that caused them to have a reaction. If your child has a reaction at school or nursery, you may feel guilty because you weren't there to protect them. These are perfectly normal feelings but remember that you would never do anything to hurt your child on purpose. Everyone makes mistakes – we are all only human. No one can watch their child every minute of the day, and nor should they!

Build a support network. Friends and family can give you general support. You will need people you can talk to, and also people who can offer practical help like looking after siblings while you attend medical appointments, or collecting prescriptions for you. You can also connect with other allergy parents through social media and online groups.

Difficult situations will arise at times. Use problem-solving strategies to try and deal with the issue. Dedicate some time to sit down and think about your particular worries and plan what you need to do, and when you are going to do it. You might find it helpful to write down all the possible solutions, to help you choose the best one for you. This is much more effective than letting worries go round and round in your head.

Sometimes, there will be nothing you can do about a problem. At these times remember that you can still control your reaction to the issue in question. Practice acceptance and self-compassion. This doesn't mean that you are happy about it, but that you recognise that you can't do anything about it at the moment. Struggling against a situation that you cannot change will only increase your suffering.

After a while, food allergies will become your new 'normal' and you will feel confident that you can manage your child's allergies safely. There are still steps that you have to take every day to keep your child safe, but you have a routine, you know which foods are safe, and there is less uncertainty. Once in a while something will happen that can rock the boat such as:

- An accidental reaction.
- Developing new allergies or co-existing conditions such as asthma or eczema.
- Learning new and conflicting information about allergies from different sources.
- Repeat testing.
- Oral food challenges in hospital.
- Food reintroduction at home.
- Developmental changes as your child begins to understand the full repercussions of their condition.
- Transitions such as starting nursery or school.
- Overnight stays away from home such as sleepovers or school trips.

During stressful periods, prioritise relaxation time. You may feel you are too busy or have too many worries to relax, but you will be much more able to cope with what life throws at you if you take time to recharge your batteries. This can be as little as 10 minutes a day (although the more stressed you are, the longer you should spend). Stress relief is very personal, but in general it just means doing something you enjoy and find relaxing. Here are some simple ideas:

- Practise deep breathing, focusing on extending the exhalation.
- Have a bubble bath with relaxing music.
- Write down your feelings in a journal.
- Go for a walk.
- Listen to your favourite songs. Even better, get dancing!
- Use a mindfulness or meditation app.
- Play a sport.

- Watch a favourite movie.
- Gardening.
- Be creative – drawing, painting, doodling, scrapbooking, photography etc.

YOUR CHILD'S EMOTIONS

If your child was diagnosed with allergies at an early age, then it will feel normal to them to have eat different things to other people and take extra precautions around food. However, they will experience new situations as they grow up that bring new challenges for them.

If your child is diagnosed with allergies at an older age, then they may feel a sense of loss at the foods they are no longer allowed to eat. They may also feel anxious and uncertain of what they should do to keep safe, but this will decrease over time as they learn more about it.

When talking to your child about their allergies keep it low key. Don't make them scared of their food allergen. At some point they may be able to reintroduce it, or need to do a food challenge, which is more difficult if they are too afraid to eat it. You will need to talk to them many times over the years to educate them about food allergies. It is an ongoing process. Keep it age-appropriate. For example:

- A toddler might understand 'You're not allowed [certain food].'
- A pre-schooler might understand 'If you eat [certain food], it makes you feel poorly.'
- A primary school child might understand 'Your body thinks [certain food] is bad and tries to get rid of it.'
- A teenager might begin to understand what anaphylaxis is and that it can be fatal.

Set clear boundaries around food and stick to them. Talk to them in the same way you would about crossing the road safely. Start from a young age so it becomes habit. For example:

- Always check with a parent before accepting food from someone else.
- Never swap food with friends.
- Always carry your epinephrine/asthma inhaler with you.
- Always wash your hands before you eat.

There are times that may bring up difficult feelings for your child. For example, if they 'fail' an allergy blood test, skin prick test or food challenge they may feel disappointment. You can't always anticipate everything and they may end up left out of some situations due to their allergy. Sometimes young children can tease others about the things that make them different – this is usually due to a lack of understanding of how this makes the person feel.

Point out other people with food allergies or restricted diets. It's not uncommon these days and your child will feel less alone if they know others are going through the same thing. Show them all the wonderful new free from foods that are being sold especially for people just like them. Explain that we are all different – life would be very boring if we were all the same! Everyone has problems and difficulties to overcome.

If your doctor advises you to start reintroducing the food, they may feel confused at first – why are you suddenly asking them to eat a food that you've always told them will make them feel ill? It may take them some time get used to this idea before they feel ready to actually eat the food, depending on their age and circumstances.

Your child does need to learn to be careful around food, but there must be a balance. If they are overly cautious they may become anxious and avoid doing things they want to do. Recognise when they are doing a good job of keeping themselves safe, and then work on the worries that are getting in the way. Give your child plenty of opportunities to talk about their feelings, any difficulties they may be having and anything they are worried about. Don't dismiss their thoughts or offer empty reassurance that 'you'll be fine'. Ask them 'What are you afraid of?'. Challenge negative thoughts – are they logical? What would you do in that situation? Teach them problem-solving strategies. Ensure they have plenty of down time to relax and play.

If your child suddenly feels more anxious than usual, make sure they understand their food allergy properly. It may be that they are entering a new developmental phase, are able to understand more, and need more information. If necessary take your child back to the doctor to discuss it with them.

Teach your child about anxiety if you feel it is becoming a problem. The physical symptoms of anxiety can be similar to those of an allergic reaction, which can cause further anxiety, so be sure your child understands the difference between the two. Monitor any particular situations that trigger anxiety so you can take action. Discuss relaxation techniques such as deep breathing, muscle relaxation and positive visualisation.

Make sure your child builds a sense of self that does not revolve around food allergies and what they cannot do. Give them lots of chances to do things they love. Encourage them to have lots of interests and plenty of friends.

It is normal for children to experience a wide spectrum of emotions at different ages and stages but keep an eye on them. Talk to other parents with similar age children to get an idea of 'normal' behaviours. Seek help if you are still concerned. Here are some things to look out for, and if you are worried, seek professional help:

- Sudden and/or dramatic changes in behaviour.
- Suddenly not eating at school (or another location).
- Eating less at home.
- Suddenly not wanting to go to school (or another location).
- Refusing to eat foods they are not allergic to because they are nervous of a reaction.
- Avoiding doing things they usually enjoy.
- If your child seems sad, withdrawn, angry or frustrated for a long period of time.

Remember that there are positives too. Children who experience adversity in childhood often grow up knowing how to deal with challenges better than their peers. They will have more empathy for others and will be more responsible. They often end up being great advocates for other people, especially others with food allergies.

The emotional aspects of living with food allergy are often overlooked. Even for families where the child's food allergy is well-controlled, there can be a huge amount of stress. This is due to the amount of extra planning and preparation involved, having to be cautious around food, and anxiety about the risk of a reaction. Don't forget to take care of your child's emotional health, as well as your own.

KEY POINTS

- Food allergies places an emotional burden on families.
- Take care of your family's emotional needs.
- Get as much help and support as you can.
- Your family will adjust to living with allergies but there will be certain times in life that increase uncertainty.
- Give your child opportunities to talk about their feelings around having food allergies.

REFERENCES AND LINKS

- Antolín-Amérigo, D, Manso, L, Caminati, M, de la Hoz Caballer, B, Cerecedo, I, Muriel, A, Rodríguez-Rodríguez, M, Barbarroja-Escudero, J, José Sánchez-González, M, Huertas-Barbudo, B, and Alvarez-MonDario, M, 'Quality of life in patients with food allergy' *Clinical and Molecular Allergy*, 14, 4 (2016) doi: [10.1186/s12948-016-0041-4].
- Esselman, Mary and Smith, Gwen, 'Allergy's High Anxiety: How To Tame Kids' Fears Of Food Reactions' *Allergic Living* (July 2016), https://www.allergicliving.com/2016/07/16/allergys-high-anxiety-tame-kids-fears-food-reactions/, accessed 11th December 2018.
- Herbert, Linda, 'Psychosocial Aspects Of Food Allergy Among Adolescents' [video], *Food Allergy Research and*

Education (2016),
https://www.youtube.com/watch?v=m1eqL_wSVJI,
accessed 11th December 2018.

- The New Indian Express, 'Kids With Chronic Asthma,
  Food Allergies At Risk Of Developing Mental Health
  Problems' (January 2018),
  http://www.newindianexpress.com/lifestyle/health/2018
  /jan/06/kids-with-chronic-asthma-food-allergies-at-risk-
  of-developing-mental-health-problems-1746074.html,
  accessed 11th December 2018.

CHAPTER 16

USEFUL LINKS AND RESOURCES

UK ALLERGY CHARITIES

Allergy UK – the leading national charity providing support for those with allergies.
Website: https://www.allergyuk.org/
Helpline: 01322 619898

Anaphylaxis Campaign – supporting people at risk of severe allergies
Website: https://www.anaphylaxis.org.uk/
Helpline: 01252 542029

Asthma UK
Website: https://www.asthma.org.uk/
Helpline: 0300 222 5800

CMPA Support – Support for the day to day management of Cow's Milk and Multiple Food Protein Allergies in Infancy and Childhood
Website: http://cowsmilkproteinallergysupport.webs.com/

FABED – Families Affected by Eosiniphilic Disorders
Website: http://www.fabed.co.uk/

FPIES Foundation
Website: http://fpiesfoundation.org/ (US website)

FPIES UK (Food Protein Induced Enterocolitis Syndrome)
Website: https://www.fpiesuk.org/

National Eczema Society
Website: http://www.eczema.org/
Helpline: 0800 089 1122 or email helpline@eczema.org

OTHER WEBSITES

Allerglobal – free, basic, personalised translation cards for travelling abroad.
http://www.allerglobal.com/

Allergy Action Translation Cards – free, detailed, personalised translation cards for travelling abroad.
https://allergyaction.org/translations/

Allergy Diner – UK restaurant reviews by people with food allergies.
https://www.allergydiner.com/

Allergic Living – online magazine for all types of allergies.
http://www.allergicliving.com (US website)

Allergy Travels – reviews of countries and airlines by people with food allergies.
https://allergytravels.com/

Food Standards Agency: Report a Food Problem – report a business that is not meeting food allergy laws or food hygiene standards.
https://www.food.gov.uk/contact/consumers/report-problem

ABOUT THE AUTHOR

Zoe T. Williams is a former adult education tutor, mother of two, and food allergy blogger at *My Allergy Kitchen*. In 2014, her youngest daughter was born. By 1 year of age she had developed six food allergies to milk, soya, wheat, eggs, oats and legumes. Zoe spent countless hours researching food allergies online: reading websites and blogs, studying journal articles, watching videos and asking questions on support forums. In this book she shares everything she has learned over the past four years, to help others going through the same journey.

Zoe is passionate about supporting parents of children with food allergies, as well as raising awareness and changing public attitudes towards food allergy.

Visit the author online at www.myallergykitchen.com.